Recognition and Treatment of Psychiatric Disorders

A Psychopharmacology Handbook for Primary Care

Charles B. Nemeroff, MD, PhD
Reunette W. Harris Professor and Chairman
Department of Psychiatry and Behavioral Sciences
Emory University School of Medicine
Atlanta, Georgia

Alan F. Schatzberg, MD
Kenneth T. Norris, Jr Professor in Psychiatry and
  Behavioral Sciences
Chairman, Department of Psychiatry and
  Behavioral Sciences
Stanford University School of Medicine
Stanford, California

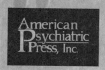
American Psychiatric Press, Inc.

Washington, DC
London, England

First Edition
Copyright © 1999 American Psychiatric Press, Inc.
02 01 00 99   4 3 2 1
ALL RIGHTS RESERVED
Manufactured in the United States of America on acid-free paper

American Psychiatric Press, Inc.
1400 K Street, NW
Washington, DC 20005
www.appi.org

Library of Congress Cataloging-in-Publication Data
Nemeroff, Charles B.
         Recognition and treatment of psychiatric disorders : a
psychopharmacology handbook for primary care / Charles B. Nemeroff,
Alan F. Schatzberg ; 1st ed.
            p.   cm.
         Includes bibliographical references and index.
         ISBN 0-88048-990-1
            1. Mental illness—Treatment Handbooks, manuals, etc.
2. Psychopharmacology Handbooks, manuals, etc.   3. Primary care
(Medicine) Handbooks, manuals, etc.   I. Schatzberg, Alan F.
II. Title.
         [DNLM: 1. Mental Disorders—drug therapy Handbooks.   2. Mental
Disorders—diagnosis Handbooks.   3. Psychotropic Drugs Handbooks.
WM 34 N433r 1999]
RC454.4.N46 1999
616.89'.18—dc21
DNLM/DLC
for Library of Congress   99-15420
                                                                                                     CIP

British Library Cataloguing in Publication Data
A CIP record is available from the British Library.

Table of Contents

Preface

Mental health is an important public health issue, as evidenced by the prevalence of psychiatric problems that are associated with tremendous disability, immense personal suffering, and a heavy economic burden.[1,2] National survey data indicate that 48% of a representative US adult sample population have reported a psychiatric disorder at one time or another and that about 30% have reported a disorder during the past 12 months. Less than half of those with a lifetime history of a psychiatric disorder ever received treatment. Interestingly, 14% of the sample reported a lifetime history of three or more comorbid psychiatric disorders.[3] These findings speak directly to the importance of screening, identifying, and treating patients with mental illness.

The primary care setting has been called a *de facto mental healthcare system* in the US[4] and the *hidden mental health network*.[5] About 60% of patients with a psychiatric disorder are identified and receive treatment in a primary care setting.[4] With the changing healthcare environment in the US, more and more patients are entering the primary care network, creating ever larger, busier, and more closely regulated practices. Thus, primary care physicians are being forced to develop or refine strategies for screening and identifying patients with psychiatric disorders.

This handbook, *Recognition and Treatment of Psychiatric Disorders: A Psychopharmacology Handbook for Primary Care*, was developed to address these issues and meet some of these needs. Another factor that led to the development of this handbook is the continually growing number of new drugs being introduced for the treatment of mental disorders and of currently available drugs being used for new psychiatric indications. Although many psychiatric disorders are suitable for treatment in the primary care setting, issues for referral to psychiatric colleagues are germane to contemporary practice and are discussed in this text. We recognize that primary care physicians have little extra time to read the voluminous psychiatric literature and distill it down to practical yet timely and accurate treatment strategies, and we hope this handbook will aid in that endeavor.

We thank SmithKline Beecham Pharmaceuticals for providing an unrestricted educational grant to Scientific Therapeutics Information, Inc, for the development of this handbook. The editorial assistance of Diane M. Coniglio, PharmD, and the staff of Scientific Therapeutics Information, Inc, is gratefully acknowledged. We also appreciate the support of our publisher, American Psychiatric Press, Inc.

Charles B. Nemeroff, MD, PhD   Alan F. Schatzberg, MD

Introduction

This handbook was designed to provide primary care physicians with brief, practical information on the pharmacologic treatment of common psychiatric disorders in adults. The handbook has two main sections. "Overview and Pharmacotherapy of Psychiatric Disorders" provides a short description of the epidemiology, pathophysiology, presentation, diagnostic criteria, and screening tests for common psychiatric disorders that may be seen in a primary care setting. This section also contains treatment algorithms and other step-by-step approaches to direct the primary care physician. "Psychopharmacologic Agents" reviews basic pharmacology, pharmacokinetics, drug interaction and safety concerns, and practical dosing issues for all classes of drugs used to treat mental disorders. Also included is a glossary of terms and abbreviations, a listing of printed or electronic mental health resources, a bibliography of all cited references, and an appendix containing selected diagnostic rating scales.

We hope this format will make the handbook easy to use and informative for primary care physicians. We welcome your comments.

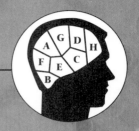

Overview and Pharmacotherapy of Psychiatric Disorders

Anxiety Disorders

Anxiety disorders are the most common psychiatric conditions in the US, with approximately one fourth of the population overall and as many as 20% of the elderly population reporting a lifetime history of at least one anxiety disorder.[3,6] Anxiety disorders are nearly twice as common in women and are more common in low- to middle-income brackets and education levels.[3] Anxiety disorders often coexist with depression,[7] especially in primary care settings, making diagnosis more difficult, treatment more complicated, and prognosis less favorable.

PANIC DISORDER

Panic disorder (PD) is a chronic but treatable problem, fraught with a high degree of social and work impairment, poor quality of life, and frequent relapses when drug treatment or psychotherapy is withdrawn. Often unrecognized, it is associated with excessive use of medical services (especially emergency room and primary care visits). PD can occur with or without agoraphobia, which is an intense, irrational fear of being alone in places or situations (eg, driving, traveling, stores, crowds, restaurants, elevators) where escape might not be possible or, if a panic attack developed, help might not be available.

Epidemiology

The lifetime prevalence of PD is between 1.5% and 3.5%, but may be as high as 21% in primary care settings.[8,9] Related panic states (eg, fearful spells, panic attacks) probably occur in as many as 16% of persons during their lifetimes.[10] Although most individuals with agoraphobia also have PD, agoraphobia can occur independently. Agoraphobia is more common in women and is the second most common anxiety disorder in the elderly.[6]

PD is twice as common in women[3,11] and is the least common anxiety disorder in the elderly.[6] There is a genetic component to PD; first-degree relatives have a four to seven times greater risk of developing PD.[12,13] This disorder typically appears between late adolescence and the mid 30s; onset in childhood or after age 45 is rare but possible. PD often is comorbid with depression, other anxiety disorders, or substance abuse.[14] Comorbidity predicts a worse prognosis for the patient with PD and has implications for drug treatment. Although the frequency of individual panic attacks varies widely among patients, syndromal PD is a chronic condition in which fear and avoidant behavior are often persistent.

Pathophysiology

- Probably caused by combined dysregulation of serotonergic, noradrenergic, γ-aminobutyric acid (GABA), dopaminergic, and brain cholecystokinin (CCK) neurotransmitter systems[15,16]

- Agents that primarily ↑ serotonergic transmission (eg, selective serotonin reuptake inhibitors [SSRIs], clomipramine) or potentiate GABA (eg, benzodiazepines) are most effective

- Agents with primarily noradrenergic activity (eg, desipramine) may be effective for some patients, but data from controlled clinical trials are lacking.[15]

Presentation

A patient with PD must have at least some spontaneous panic attacks (ie, a discrete, intense period of sudden apprehension, fearfulness, or terror possibly associated with a feeling of impending doom),[12,13] anticipatory and generalized anxiety, agoraphobia (see below), somatic symptoms (Table 1), and obsessions.[17] Somatic symptoms often are misinterpreted as nonpsychiatric medical conditions (and the converse is true, also). Approximately one half of individuals with PD have agoraphobia.[10]

Table 1. Common symptoms of panic attack[12,13]

- Palpitations, pounding heart, ↑ heart rate
- Sweating
- Choking feeling
- Nausea or abdominal distress
- Feelings of being detached from oneself (depersonalization) or unreality (derealization)
- Fear of dying
- Feelings of losing control

- Shortness of breath, smothering feeling
- Chest pain, discomfort
- Trembling, shaking
- Numbness, tingling
- Feeling dizzy, light-headed, faint
- Chills or hot flashes

Diagnosis/Screening Tools

Diagnosing PD can be difficult because presenting physical symptoms often mimic other medical conditions (eg, angina, dyspepsia).[18] The Sheehan Patient Rated Anxiety Scale or the MINI (Parts E and F; see APPENDIX) may be useful in the primary care setting. Commonly, patients with unrecognized PD undergo extensive tests for nonexistent clinical diseases (eg, coronary artery disease [CAD], ulcer disease) and are frequent users of the emergency department, primary care office, and specialists.[18] By understanding the common presentations of PD, the primary care physician can screen patients for PD and interrupt the costly and often unnecessary utilization of healthcare services.

A diagnosis of a panic attack is made when four or more cognitive or physical symptoms (Table 1) occur during a spontaneous and discrete period of intense fear or discomfort; symptoms must reach peak intensity within 10 minutes.[11] Panic attacks may be *unexpected* (ie, spontaneous, not associated with a trigger), *situationally bound* (ie, occurring immediately on exposure to or anticipation of a trigger), or *situationally predisposed* (ie, likely to occur with exposure to a trigger but may occur later or not at all).[12,13] PD is characterized by recurrent, unexpected panic attacks, persistent worry (≥1 mo) about having another attack (anticipatory anxiety), and change in behavior because of the attacks or related anxiety.[11]

Medical conditions (eg, angina, hyperthyroidism, pheochromocytoma) or substance abuse (eg, alcohol, caffeine, cocaine) that might cause similar symptoms should be ruled out. There are no diagnostic laboratory tests, but some patients with PD have compensated respiratory alkalosis. Physical findings are unremarkable, but patients may have mildly elevated blood pressure (BP) during an attack.

Agoraphobia is diagnosed when a patient has significant anxiety about or avoidance of places or situations where escape would be difficult or embarrassing or, if panic-like symptoms were to occur, help might not be available.[12,13] Agoraphobic patients often become housebound because of their fears; unemployment due to an inability to work can become an important issue. Alternative diagnoses may be more appropriate if avoidance is limited to only a few discrete situations (eg, nongeneralized social anxiety disorder) or to a broader spectrum of performance or interactional situations (eg, GENERALIZED SOCIAL ANXIETY DISORDER) (see page 17).[12,13]

Referral

• Refer to a psychiatrist patients with comorbid psychiatric conditions (eg, especially those with suicidal tendencies), substance abuse problems, significantly impaired functioning caused by avoidant behavior, or poor response to therapy.

Treatment

Short-term treatment goals include symptom relief and initiation of psychologic intervention. Cognitive-behavioral psychotherapy with an experienced clinician is effective alone in mild, stable cases or in conjunction with drug therapy for patients who prefer this approach and who are willing to participate.[19] Pharmacologic treatment for PD includes certain antidepressants (especially SSRIs) or a high-potency benzodiazepine (Figure 1). Only paroxetine, sertraline, and alprazolam are currently approved by the US Food and Drug Administration (FDA) for PD. Benefits of long-term drug treatment are controversial but long-term therapy does appear to reduce the risk of relapse. Physicians must evaluate the dependence liability and abuse potential of benzodiazepines when considering long-term treatment.

Antidepressants: SSRIs are first-line agents because of their documented efficacy, safety, and tolerability profile.[22-27] Both tricyclic antidepressants (TCAs) and SSRIs, particularly fluoxetine, can cause a "jitteriness" syndrome (also called activation) that presents as anxiety, insomnia, agitation, and diarrhea early in the treatment course. To minimize this syndrome, which may reduce patient compliance with the regimen, one half to one third of the usual starting dose for depression (eg, paroxetine 10 mg, fluoxetine 5 mg) should be used and increased slowly over 3 or 4 weeks until a response is observed.

Figure 1. Pharmacologic treatment approach to the patient with PD (modified from references 20 and 21). Abbreviations defined in GLOSSARY.

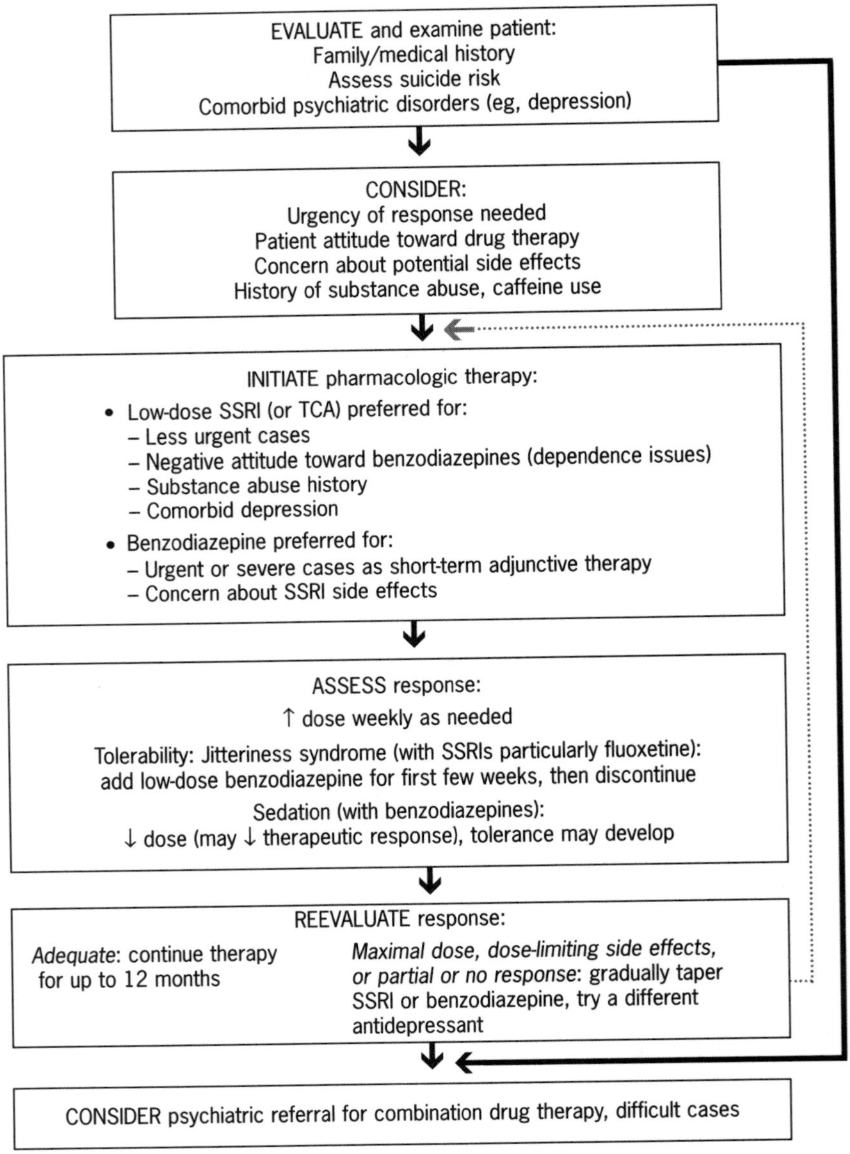

EVALUATE and examine patient:
Family/medical history
Assess suicide risk
Comorbid psychiatric disorders (eg, depression)

CONSIDER:
Urgency of response needed
Patient attitude toward drug therapy
Concern about potential side effects
History of substance abuse, caffeine use

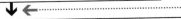

INITIATE pharmacologic therapy:

- Low-dose SSRI (or TCA) preferred for:
  - Less urgent cases
  - Negative attitude toward benzodiazepines (dependence issues)
  - Substance abuse history
  - Comorbid depression
- Benzodiazepine preferred for:
  - Urgent or severe cases as short-term adjunctive therapy
  - Concern about SSRI side effects

ASSESS response:

↑ dose weekly as needed

Tolerability: Jitteriness syndrome (with SSRIs particularly fluoxetine): add low-dose benzodiazepine for first few weeks, then discontinue

Sedation (with benzodiazepines):
↓ dose (may ↓ therapeutic response), tolerance may develop

REEVALUATE response:

Adequate: continue therapy for up to 12 months

Maximal dose, dose-limiting side effects, or partial or no response: gradually taper SSRI or benzodiazepine, try a different antidepressant

CONSIDER psychiatric referral for combination drug therapy, difficult cases

Concurrent use of a low-dose benzodiazepine also may alleviate these symptoms while the SSRI is being titrated. Long-term SSRI use can be associated with sexual dysfunction in both men and women; this concern should be discussed with the patient. With the SSRIs, a clinical response may not be noted for 3 to 6 weeks; if a rapid response is needed for severe cases, benzodiazepine therapy may be preferred. Emerging data with venlafaxine and nefazodone are promising for treatment of PD.[12,15]

Benzodiazepines: The SSRIs have largely replaced the benzodiazepines as first-line treatment of PD. High-potency benzodiazepines (eg, alprazolam, clonazepam, lorazepam) are effective at rapidly relieving anxiety. High doses are sometimes needed (eg, alprazolam up to 10 mg). Low doses should be used initially (eg, alprazolam 0.5 mg two or three times daily [BID or TID]) with subsequent dose increases as needed and tolerated. Side effects may limit the ability to increase the dose to obtain maximal benefit. Some patients are unwilling to take benzodiazepines because of dependence or tolerance issues. The primary side effect of benzodiazepine therapy is sedation, which can be reduced by lowering the dose; tolerance to this effect also may develop.

OBSESSIVE-COMPULSIVE DISORDER

Obsessions are recurrent, intrusive thoughts that are considered excessive, senseless, or repugnant by the patient and that cause significant anxiety. Compulsions are time-consuming, repetitive behaviors that neutralize or relieve the anxiety caused by obsessions[13] (Table 2).

Table 2. Common obsessions and compulsions in adults with OCD[13,28]

- Obsessions: Contamination, pathologic doubt, somatic concerns, need for symmetry or order, aggressive or sexual impulses
- Compulsions: Checking, washing, cleaning, counting, repeatedly asking or confessing, ordering (for symmetry or precision), hoarding

Abbreviations defined in GLOSSARY.

Epidemiology

Obsessive-compulsive disorder (OCD) is a chronic, relapsing illness that is more common than previously thought. It affects more than 4 million people in the US.[29,30] The lifetime prevalence of OCD is 2% to 3%; the disorder is equally common in men and women.[31] A genetic component has not been firmly established, but anxiety disorders in general are more common among relatives of patients with OCD[32] and there may be a genetic link between OCD and Tourette's syndrome. Frequently, OCD is comorbid with depression, other anxiety disorders (eg, simple phobia or social anxiety disorder, PD), personality disorders, or alcohol abuse.[28] Other obsessive behaviors such as trichotillomania (hair pulling), compulsive gambling, compulsive sexual behaviors, or eating disorders may be related to OCD.[30]

Pathophysiology

- Abnormal serotonin regulation,[33] although dopamine and neuropeptides also may be involved.[32]

Presentation

The onset of OCD usually occurs before age 25; a large proportion of cases begin in childhood.[30] Patients with OCD usually display both obsessions and compulsions (Table 2), which can become a significant source of embarrassment, depending on the level of insight a patient has into his or her symptoms. A typical presentation of OCD is germ obsession with handwashing. Patients tend to seek help when their behavior can no longer be hidden from nonfamily members or becomes significantly disruptive to their lives. Typically, several years elapse between the onset of symptoms and seeking medical help. Therefore, guilt, helplessness, and loss of self-esteem at being unable to hide the condition are common presenting symptoms. Precipitating factors include sexual or marital problems, pregnancy, childbirth,[34] and death or illness of a close relative.[30] OCD is a chronic illness; in about 50% of cases, the course is continual whereas in others, symptom severity fluctuates. Patients with a previously normal personality, an episodic course, and a short illness may fare better than those with an obsessional premorbid personality, severe illness at presentation, unmarried status, or childhood nervousness.[30]

Diagnosis/Screening Tools

The Florida Yale-Brown Obsessive Compulsive Scale (FLY-BOCS; see APPENDIX) or the MINI (Part H; see APPENDIX) can be used to identify symptoms of OCD and monitor response to therapy.[35] Diagnostic criteria are provided in Table 3.[13] Several psychiatric disorders (eg, personality disorders, hypochondriasis, depression, schizophrenia, phobias, and Tourette's syndrome) share clinical features of OCD and should be ruled out.[13,28,30] Comorbid psychiatric disorders also should be identified. There are no diagnostic tests for OCD; dermatologic conditions caused by excessive washing may be evident in some patients.

Referral

- Refer patients to a trained psychotherapist for adjunctive cognitive-behavioral therapy (CBT); this important and effective component may improve long-term outcome[30]

- Consider psychiatric referral if other mental disorders are present or if patient is severely incapacitated, unable to work, leave the house, or expresses suicidal ideation.

Table 3. Diagnostic criteria for OCD in adults (adapted from reference 13, with permission). © Copyright 1994, American Psychiatric Association.

- Either obsessions or compulsions:
  - obsessions: recurrent, persistent thoughts, impulses or images (see Table 2) that are intrusive, inappropriate, and cause marked anxiety or distress, and that are not excessive worries about real-life problems; attempts are made to ignore, suppress, or neutralize them with another action, and patient recognizes that the behaviors are a product of his or her mind
  - compulsions: repetitive behaviors or mental acts (see Table 2) performed in response to obsessions and aimed at preventing or reducing distress
- Patient recognizes behaviors as excessive and unreasonable
- Behaviors must cause marked distress and be time consuming (>1 h/d) or significantly interfere with occupational, social, and family or intimate relationships

Abbreviations defined in GLOSSARY.

Treatment

An individualized treatment regimen incorporating behavioral,[36] psychosocial, and pharmacologic approaches is necessary to relieve acute symptoms of OCD and prevent relapse (Figure 2). For mild OCD, behavioral intervention is preferred for initial treatment; however, for moderate to severe cases, drug treatment also is indicated.[39]

For more than 20 years, the TCA clomipramine has been the benchmark pharmacologic treatment.[40,41] Because it has specific activity at serotonin reuptake sites, clomipramine is far more effective than other TCAs that preferentially block norepinephrine reuptake (eg, nortriptyline, desipramine) (see Table 41). By the same token, SSRIs (see page 82) are highly effective in OCD and are now considered by many to be first-line treatment because of greater tolerability and safety in overdose.[26,38,39,42]

Initial doses of SSRIs or clomipramine (Table 4) should be titrated slowly upward as tolerated. Doses needed for the treatment of OCD may be higher than for other anxiety disorders or for depression. Patients should be advised that clinical response may be delayed for 6 weeks or more. A 10- to 12-week therapeutic trial should be attempted at a maximal tolerated dose before nonresponse is considered.

Switching to another SSRI or using clomipramine may benefit nonresponders. However, in the 30% of patients who do not respond to monotherapy, combination treatment may be tried, although the benefits of this approach are not clear.[37,38] Buspirone can be added to SSRI therapy for anxious patients (alone, buspirone is of little benefit); trazodone also may be useful with an SSRI. Other agents that may be effective when added to SSRI or clomipramine therapy include clonazepam, antipsychotics (in patients with delusions or tics), or lithium.[37,38] Full-dose drug therapy should be maintained for at least 1 year in responders and behavioral intervention used to reduce the risk of relapse.[17] In a long-term paroxetine maintenance study, patients who discontinued medication therapy had a risk of relapse that was 2.7 times greater than patients who remained on therapy.[43]

Figure 2. Pharmacologic treatment approach to the patient with OCD.[37-39] Abbreviations defined in GLOSSARY.

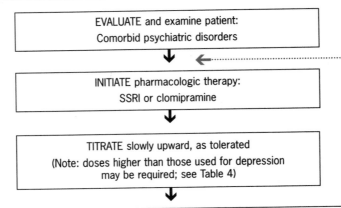

EVALUATE and examine patient:
Comorbid psychiatric disorders

↓ ←

INITIATE pharmacologic therapy:
SSRI or clomipramine

↓

TITRATE slowly upward, as tolerated
(Note: doses higher than those used for depression
may be required; see Table 4)

↓

ASSESS response after 4 - 6 weeks, tolerability:

Full: Continue drug for at least 1 year; gradually taper (↓ 25% every 2 months)

Partial: ↑ Dose to maximum, switch to alternate SSRI or clomipramine, or consider combination treatment with buspirone (comorbid anxiety), lithium, clonazepam, antipsychotic (comorbid delusions, tics), or alternate antidepressant (eg, trazodone)

None: Try alternate SSRI (as above) or clomipramine; consider psychiatric referral

CONSIDER psychiatric referral for CBT or for difficult or nonresponding cases

Table 4. Dosing strategies for clomipramine and SSRIs in OCD[38,39]

Drug	Dose (mg/d)	
	Initial	Maximal
Clomipramine	25 - 50	250 - 300
Fluoxetine	10 - 20	60 - 80
Fluvoxamine	50	300
Paroxetine	20	60
Sertraline	50	200 - 225

Abbreviations defined in GLOSSARY.

POSTTRAUMATIC STRESS DISORDER

Posttraumatic stress disorder (PTSD) is an anxiety disorder that develops after a specific or repeated life-threatening stressor or traumatic event such as sexual abuse, torture, criminal activity (either directed at the patient or that the patient witnessed), automobile accident, burn injury, or war.

Epidemiology

The lifetime prevalence of PTSD is between 1% and 14% but may be as high as 58% in at-risk populations (eg, combat veterans).[44,45] PTSD is chronic[46] and most cases are comorbid with substance abuse, depression, or anxiety disorders.[47-49]

Pathophysiology

- Derangements in several neurobiological systems[50]
- Serotonergic dysfunction → irritability and impulsive, aggressive symptoms[51]
- Noradrenergic, serotonergic, corticotropin-releasing factor (CRF), and dopaminergic systems may be involved in startle reactions.[50,52]

Presentation

PTSD can occur at any age. Symptoms usually begin within 3 months of the trauma (acute PTSD) but can be delayed 6 months or more after the event. Persons with war-zone-related PTSD probably differ from those with civilian-related trauma (eg, sexual assault, child abuse). Characteristic symptoms include hyperarousal (eg, being hypervigilant, easily startled) and intermittent autonomic hyperactivity (eg, elevated BP, heart rate) upon exposure or re-exposure to situations reminiscent of the original stressor.[32] Intrusive symptoms such as disrupted sleep and daytime flashbacks or vivid dreams are common. Avoidance symptoms include social withdrawal (numbing of emotions) and partial amnesia of the event. Hypothalamic-pituitary-adrenal (HPA) axis function may be abnormal.

War-zone veterans with PTSD report that alcohol and other illicit drug use (eg, marijuana, heroin) improves PTSD symptoms; thus, alcoholism and substance abuse are commonly comorbid with PTSD. In this population, PTSD may be followed first by generalized anxiety disorder (GAD) or alcoholism and later by phobias, depression, and PD.[46]

Diagnosis/Screening Tools

Diagnostic criteria for PTSD in adults (Table 5) comprise a triad of intrusive, avoidant, and hyperarousal symptoms, and all must be present to make the diagnosis.[13] The Treatment Outcome PTSD Scale (TOP-8) or the MINI (Part I) may be used to identify traumatic events and symptom severity (see APPENDIX). Screening tools/questionnaires used to evaluate war-zone veterans may not be useful in the civilian population and vice versa.[53]

Table 5. Diagnostic criteria for PTSD (adapted from reference 13, with permission). © Copyright 1994, American Psychiatric Association.

- Experiencing or witnessing a traumatic (life-threatening) event involving actual or threatened death or serious personal harm
  – response involved intense fear, helplessness, or horror
- Persistent reexperiencing of the traumatic event
  – recurrent, intrusive recollections, dreams, "flashbacks," hallucinations
- Persistent avoidance of stimuli associated with the trauma and numbed responsiveness
  – diminished interest or participation in activities, feelings of detachment or estrangement
- ≥2 persistent (>1 mo) symptoms of increased arousal
  – sleep difficulties, angry outbursts, hypervigilance, difficulty concentrating, exaggerated startle response
- Clinically significant distress/impairment in social, occupational, and other areas of functioning

Abbreviations defined in GLOSSARY.

Referral

- Refer patients with suspected or documented PTSD to a practitioner skilled in trauma-based psychotherapy.

Treatment

PTSD is often chronic; drug treatment alone is likely to provide only moderate improvement for only certain symptoms.[54] Some symptoms (eg, avoidance) may respond better to psychotherapy and permit concurrent improvement in other facets of the condition. Among the very limited data on the pharmacotherapy of PTSD, most are from studies of war-zone veterans. Unfortunately, clinical response may differ depending on the source of the trauma (ie, veterans in one study did not respond to an SSRI but civilian trauma victims did[55]). The focus of drug therapy is relief of the most distressing symptom(s) as perceived by the patient.[48] Positive symptoms (ie, intrusive or hyperarousal) may respond to drug therapy better than negative symptoms (ie, avoidance or withdrawal), but evidence shows the SSRIs to be effective for the latter as well.

Antidepressants: SSRIs offer clinical benefit and good overall tolerability and safety, making them preferred initial therapy for PTSD (Figure 3).[48,51,56] Use of low doses initially will minimize the jitteriness or anxiety symptoms that can accompany SSRI use (see page 86), but full antidepressant doses usually will be required (see Table 45). TCAs, monoamine oxidase inhibitors (MAOIs), and trazodone have shown some benefit in war veterans with PTSD and can be used if SSRIs fail.[48,57,58] A major limitation of MAOI therapy is the common comorbidity of alcohol or substance abuse and the inherent risk of hypertensive reactions.

Figure 3. Pharmacologic treatment approach to the patient with PTSD.[48] Abbreviations defined in GLOSSARY.

EVALUATE and examine patient:
Comorbid psychiatric disorders (eg, depression, PD, substance use)

↓

INITIATE pharmacologic therapy:
Low-dose SSRI

↓

ASSESS response and tolerability:

↑ SSRI dose gradually to usual antidepressant doses (see Table 45)

Full: Treat at least 6 - 12 months after symptoms remit or are reduced in severity. Consider gradual taper to discontinuation. If symptoms recur, restart therapy and continue indefinitely

Partial: Continue treatment as above. Consider adding carbamazepine, lithium, or valproic acid to reduce impulsive/aggressive behavior or intrusive symptoms

None: Confirm diagnosis. Change to another antidepressant (avoid MAOI in patients with history of alcohol or substance abuse); consider psychiatric referral

↓

CONSIDER psychiatric referral for combination drug therapy or difficult cases

The lack of clinical studies in patients with PTSD permits no conclusions to be made with regard to the ideal duration of drug therapy. However, because PTSD is often a chronic disorder, it is likely that therapy should be continued for at least 12 months; if discontinuation is desired, it should be preceded by a gradual taper.

Miscellaneous: Benzodiazepines relieve only anxiety symptoms of PTSD and are ineffective as monotherapy; they also carry significant risks of dependence and abuse.[48] ß-Blockers used with an antidepressant may reduce sympathomimetic hyperactivity. Carbamazepine, valproic acid, or lithium may reduce aggressive outbursts and can be used in conjunction with ongoing antidepressant therapy.[59]

GENERALIZED ANXIETY DISORDER

GAD is a chronic state of worry, anxiety, nervousness, or apprehension that is excessive (ie, present more days than not for ≥6 mo) and unrelated to another mood or anxiety disorder.[13]

Epidemiology

The lifetime prevalence is approximately 5%, and the disorder is twice as common in women as in men.[3,6] GAD is commonly comorbid; as many as 40% of patients with GAD have major depression.[60] Other anxiety disorders, alcohol or substance abuse, or depression also are frequent in patients with GAD. This fact not only blurs diagnostic accuracy, but also has important treatment implications.[60,61] Comorbidity is especially common in elderly patients with GAD.

Pathophysiology

- Abnormal regulation of several neurobiologic components (eg, serotonin, GABA, sympathetic nervous systems, CCK, HPA, etc) during times of stress but not typically during periods of rest.[62]

Presentation

Chronic hyperarousal and anxiety are hallmarks of GAD.[17] In addition to the diagnostic criteria (Table 6), physical symptoms (eg, sweating, cold clammy hands, chills, nausea, diarrhea, trouble swallowing ["lump in the throat"], urinary frequency) are common. Worries tend to be focused on everyday life situations such as job responsibilities, finances, health, children, or minor issues (eg, being late for an appointment). Many with GAD report being anxious all their lives; more than half seek treatment while in childhood or adolescence.[13] GAD is chronic[63] and tends to be worse during times of stress.[13] Persons with GAD commonly express signs or symptoms of depression, other anxiety disorders, or substance abuse disorders.

Table 6. Diagnostic criteria for GAD (adapted from reference 13, with permission).
© Copyright 1994, American Psychiatric Association.

- Excessive anxiety and worry occurring more days than not for ≥6 months
- Difficulty in controlling the worry
- ≥3 symptoms present
  - feeling restless or being on edge
  - being easily fatigued
  - difficulty concentrating, mind going blank
  - irritability
  - muscle tension
  - sleep disturbances (difficulty falling asleep or restless, unsatisfying sleep)
- Clinically significant impairment of social or occupational functioning
- Worry not due to substance abuse, medical condition, or to another psychiatric disorder

Abbreviations defined in GLOSSARY.

Diagnosis/Screening Tools

GAD often is a diagnosis of exclusion.[64] The MINI (Part O; see APPENDIX) may be useful as a brief structured interview. The diagnosis is made when uncontrollable anxiety or worry is accompanied by three or more symptoms (Table 6) and anxiety is not related to another psychiatric disorder (eg, PD, agitated depression) or substance abuse. Finally, the patient's anxiety and physical symptoms must cause clinically significant impairment of social, occupational, or personal functioning.[13] Appropriate laboratory and diagnostic studies must be conducted to ensure that anxiety symptoms are not caused by a general medical condition (eg, pheochromocytoma, hyperthyroidism).

Referral

- Refer patients to a trained psychotherapist for adjunctive therapy
- Consider psychiatric referral for drug treatment of comorbid depression, anxiety, or substance abuse disorders.[17]

Treatment

Psychotherapy often is effective alone for mild cases and is used in conjunction with pharmacologic therapy for more severe cases.[64] Although benzodiazepines have been the mainstay of GAD therapy, antidepressants are effective in GAD because of the high rate of comorbidity with depression.[65,66] Antidepressants are associated with a lower potential for abuse or dependence and may be better tolerated than benzodiazepines. Buspirone and venlafaxine are FDA approved for GAD.

Benzodiazepines: Benzodiazepines are effective for short-term symptom relief (Figure 4); all members of the class are equally effective, and drug selection can be based on pharmacokinetic features (see Table 68). Benzodiazepines may cause addiction and dependence; for patients with a substance or alcohol abuse history, nonbenzodiazepine drugs may be preferred.[67] Benzo-diazepines also are associated with a withdrawal syndrome (see page 116). Although GAD is a chronic, recurring disorder, the long-term benefit of benzo-diazepine therapy is controversial, although some data support it.[17] Alprazolam has been suggested to be effective in patients with underlying depression, but some data indicate that benzodiazepines may actually cause or worsen depression.[61]

Figure 4. Pharmacologic treatment approach to the patient with GAD.

EVALUATE and examine patient:
Comorbid psychiatric disorders (eg, depression)

CONSIDER:
Urgency of response needed
Previous benzodiazepine use
History of substance abuse

INITIATE pharmacologic therapy:
- Benzodiazepine (eg, diazepam, oxazepam)
  - Previous benzodiazepine use or urgent response needed
  - No previous benzodiazepine use or positive substance abuse history
- Buspirone
  - Comorbid depression
- Antidepressant (eg, imipramine, SSRI)

ASSESS response:
↑ Dose of benzodiazepine or buspirone every 2 or 3 days until symptoms resolve (may take 2 - 3 weeks with buspirone) or maximum dose reached

Full: Treat 4 - 6 months and taper dose gradually. If symptoms gradually reappear[a], restart therapy and continue indefinitely

Partial or none: Confirm diagnosis, assess comorbid diagnoses, change to another agent; consider psychiatric referral

CONSIDER psychiatric referral for combination drug therapy or difficult cases

---

[a] Immediate appearance of anxiety symptoms after benzodiazepine taper may indicate with-drawal anxiety rather than re-emergence of GAD. Abbreviations defined in GLOSSARY.

Antidepressants: Antidepressants may be useful in patients with significant depressive symptoms or in anxious patients who do not respond to benzodiazepine or buspirone therapy.[68] In doses lower than those used to treat depression, imipramine has clinically important anxiolytic effects.[69] As with buspirone, however, the onset of therapeutic benefit may be delayed for 2 or more weeks. A growing body of evidence has demonstrated that the SSRI paroxetine is effective in GAD.[64,65] MAOIs also may be effective in some patients.

Buspirone: Buspirone is effective in GAD, and advantages over benzodiazepines include less drowsiness, lower abuse potential, easier discontinuation, and no exacerbation of underlying depressive symptoms.[61,70] The onset of improvement with buspirone is somewhat slower (2 to 3 weeks) than with benzodiazepines; therefore, buspirone may be most appropriate for patients not requiring acute symptomatic relief. The initial dose is 5 mg BID with periodic increases to approximately 30 mg/d as needed. Patients who previously have responded to benzodiazepine therapy may respond less well to buspirone,[64] although patients can be switched from benzodiazepine therapy to buspirone with few complications.[66] Long-term buspirone therapy is well tolerated and efficacy is maintained.

SOCIAL ANXIETY DISORDER

Social anxiety disorder (also known as social phobia), a chronic, disabling condition characterized by an intense fear of embarrassment and humiliation when observed by others, has only recently become the focus of psychiatric research. Social anxiety disorder can be generalized or nongeneralized (Table 7).

Table 7. Social anxiety disorder subtypes[71]

Subtype	Symptoms	Related impairment	Treatment
Nongeneralized	Predictable, occasional symptoms; limited to one or a few public situations (eg, speaking)	Minor	β-Blocker (eg, propranolol) or benzodiazepine PRN to diminish performance anxiety
Generalized	Most or all performance or interactional situations produce anxiety	Severe	Antidepressant or benzodiazepine needed; often treatment-resistant

Abbreviations defined in GLOSSARY.

Epidemiology

Social anxiety disorder is the most common anxiety disorder and the third most common psychiatric disorder in the US, preceded only by depression and alcohol dependence.[3] The lifetime prevalence may be as high as 13%; it is only slightly more common in women.[3,72,73] Two out of three patients with social anxiety disorder have the more disabling and difficult-to-treat generalized form.[74] The onset of social anxiety disorder usually occurs between the ages of 12 and 16 years,[75] but inhibited behavior or social anxiety that later may develop into social anxiety disorder can begin in childhood or early adolescence. Limited evidence suggests a genetic component to social anxiety disorder.[76] Persons with social anxiety disorder tend to have lower levels of education and socioeconomic status.[75] Comorbidity with other anxiety disorders, mood disorders (eg, depression), and substance abuse is common. People with social anxiety disorder with comorbid psychiatric conditions have high rates of suicidal ideation and suicide attempts.[75]

Pathophysiology

- Generalized and nongeneralized subtypes may not share a common pathophysiology
- Dopaminergic and serotonergic systems likely involved[77]
- Normal hypothalamic-pituitary-thyroid (HPT) and HPA axis function[32] and ↓ metabolic activity in certain brain areas[77]
- Only unique finding is ↑ mean arterial pressure following thyrotropin-releasing hormone (TRH) infusion.[77]

Presentation

In social situations (Table 8), patients may experience tachycardia, tremor, blushing, sweating, shortness of breath, and gastrointestinal (GI) disturbances (eg, diarrhea). The symptoms themselves or anxiety about them causes humiliation and embarrassment, which further increases discomfort. Physical and cognitive features subsequently lead to behavior such as "freezing," in which the patient is unable to function in public. Ultimately, the patient avoids such anxiety-causing situations or endures them with great discomfort.

Patients with social anxiety disorder feel guilt and shame, and have an exaggerated sense of the impact of their social performance. They recognize these feelings as irrational and therefore have low self-esteem. Their personality type may be shy or avoidant; they make poor eye contact and may have cold, clammy hands and a tremulous voice. They report substantial impairment in work, school, and social activities and are likely to be more frequent utilizers of medical services and welfare or disability than persons without social anxiety disorder.[78]

Diagnosis/Screening Tools

Social anxiety disorder is underdiagnosed (Table 9) in primary care, and patients often do not see a physician until secondary disorders (eg, depression, substance abuse) develop.

Table 8. Common fears and sources of avoidance in social anxiety disorder

- Public speaking or performance
- Eating or writing in public (eg, signing a check)
- Using public restrooms
- Being the center of attention or being stared at
- Dating
- Going to a party
- Speaking to authority figures (eg, employer, sales clerk)
- Meeting strangers

Table 9. Diagnostic criteria for social anxiety disorder (adapted from reference 13, with permission). © Copyright 1994, American Psychiatric Association.

- Marked, persistent fear of social/performance situations in which the person is subject to possible scrutiny. The person fears showing anxiety or behaving in a way that causes embarrassment or humiliation
- Exposure to the situation causes significant anxiety that may resemble a panic attack; such situations are avoided or endured with tremendous anxiety
- Fears are recognized by the patient as excessive or unreasonable. Avoidance or anxiety causes significant interference with normal functioning

Social anxiety disorder shares many features of PD, but in the former, fears are related to public performance and subsequent perception of that performance (Table 10).

Table 10. Questions to aid in making a differential diagnosis of social anxiety disorder[79]

Question	Yes	No
Can you go to a public place (eg, shopping mall) alone, without speaking to anyone?	Social anxiety disorder	Agoraphobia
Does anxiety occur when you are alone?	PD	Social anxiety disorder
Is the anxiety restricted to your performance in a social situation?	Social anxiety disorder	GAD, PD

Abbreviations defined in GLOSSARY.

The Liebowitz Social Anxiety Scale (see APPENDIX) is helpful for measuring the severity of fearful behavior and for monitoring response to treatment.[80] The Brief Social Anxiety Disorder Scale,[79] the Fear Questionnaire,[81] or the MINI (Part G; see APPENDIX) may also aid in assessing symptom severity.

Referral

- Referral for CBT, especially early after diagnosis, can be effective in treating some patients with social anxiety disorder.

Treatment

For generalized social anxiety disorder, antidepressant or benzodiazepine therapy is preferred (Figure 5). Currently, only one antidepressant (paroxetine) is FDA approved for the treatment of social anxiety disorder.

Antidepressants: A growing body of evidence supports the use of SSRIs as first-line therapy for generalized social anxiety disorder because of favorable efficacy, safety, and tolerability profiles.[26,71,82-85] In one large study, 77% of patients responded to paroxetine therapy compared with 42% of patients treated with placebo (Paxil® prescribing information, 1999). To date, the most extensive efficacy experience among the SSRIs has been with paroxetine. Usual antidepressant doses can be used unless the patient has comorbid PD; in this case, lower initial doses should be used to avoid the jitteriness that can accompany some SSRIs (see page 86). Little is known about the ideal duration of treatment, but it probably should be at least 6 months after the maximum clinical response has been reached.[71] Therapy should be gradually discontinued and restarted upon evidence of relapse. One controlled trial demonstrated that rates of relapse were significantly lower in patients whose SSRI therapy (ie, paroxetine) was maintained as compared with those whose therapy was stopped.[84] SSRIs are especially useful when social anxiety disorder is comorbid with depression, OCD, or PD.

MAOIs (eg, phenelzine) are very well studied and are effective in generalized social anxiety disorder.[86] Although less effective than MAOIs and not consistently effective in controlled trials, buspirone may be useful in patients with comorbid alcohol dependence who are not candidates for MAOIs or benzodiazepines. TCAs have not been well studied for this indication. Some evidence from uncontrolled trials and case reports suggests that both venlafaxine and nefazodone may be effective.

Benzodiazepines: High-potency, long-acting agents (eg, clonazepam) effectively reduce anxiety but dependence issues need to be considered. Rates of relapse after benzodiazepine discontinuation are high.[87]

Figure 5. Pharmacologic treatment approach to the patient with generalized social anxiety disorder.[71]

EVALUATE and examine patient:

Establish subtype: generalized or nongeneralized

Comorbid psychiatric disorders (eg, depression, PD, alcohol abuse)

INITIATE pharmacologic therapy:

Nongeneralized subtype: benzodiazepine or β-blocker PRN

Generalized subtype: SSRI in usual antidepressant doses (eg, paroxetine 20 mg) (Table 45). If PD present or suspected, use lower doses and ↑ gradually to usual antidepressant doses

ASSESS response and tolerability:

Full: Continue SSRI for 6 - 12 months after symptoms remit or are reduced in severity. Consider gradual taper to discontinuation. If symptoms recur, restart therapy and continue indefinitely

Partial: Consider adding benzodiazepine (clonazepam) or buspirone to SSRI

None: Confirm diagnosis. Assess substance abuse history; if none, use benzodiazepine (eg, clonazepam) and if present, use buspirone. Use with antidepressant if comorbid major depression or OCD; consider psychiatric referral

REASSESS response:

None: Use buspirone or MAOI[a]; consider psychiatric referral

Partial: Add buspirone or MAOI to clonazepam

CONSIDER psychiatric referral for combination drug therapy or difficult cases

[a] MAOIs should never be combined with SSRIs because of the risk of serotonin syndrome. Abbreviations defined in GLOSSARY.

Mood Disorders

Primary mood disorders include depressive disorders (eg, major [unipolar] depression, dysthymic disorder) and bipolar disorders (including mania). This section focuses on adult depression; brief sections on adolescent depression and depression in the elderly also are included for completeness.

MAJOR DEPRESSIVE DISORDER

Depression is a common, chronic, relapsing disorder associated with substantial morbidity, mortality, and excessive use of healthcare services.[88,89] Even with the multitude of effective and safe treatments, depression is frequently misdiagnosed or not diagnosed at all, especially in the busy primary care setting, which leads to either incorrect treatment or undertreatment (Table 11).[90,91] In the US, the annual cost of depression is at least $43 billion, the bulk of which is for indirect losses due to premature death, absenteeism, and reduced work productivity. These costs are similar to those for CAD and far greater than those of many other chronic illnesses such as chronic lung disease.[91]

Table 11. Reasons for the undertreatment of depression[91]

Group	Factors
Patients	Lack of recognition of depressive symptoms, ↑ focus on somatic complaints, lack of appreciation for potential severity of untreated depression, limited access to care, poor compliance with therapy, stigma of diagnosis
Providers	Lack of education about depression and available treatments or resources; poor interpersonal skills for dealing with emotional disorders; ↑ time needed to diagnose depression; lack of objective, clinical markers
Healthcare system	Inadequate insurance reimbursement for mental disorders, lack of trained psychotherapists, poor referral programs in managed care systems

Epidemiology

Up to 10% of patients in primary care settings have major depression.[92] The lifetime risk of developing depression is as high as 25% in women and 13% in men;[3] interestingly, risk factors for depression (Table 12) do not include education, income, or marital status.

Table 12. Risk factors for depression[90]

• Prior depressive episodes	• Prior suicide attempts
• Family history of depression	• Female gender (unipolar depression)
• Age <40 years at onset	• Recent childbirth
• Medical comorbidity	• Lack of social support
• Stressful life events	• Current substance abuse

Depression can start at any age but most commonly begins in individuals between the ages of 20 and 45. Major depressive disorder is three times more common in first-degree affected relatives.[93] An average untreated depressive episode lasts about 6 months. Up to 60% of patients with a single depressive episode will develop a second episode. When symptoms remit, patients usually return to a presymptomatic level of functioning. However, symptoms not meeting full diagnostic criteria can persist for months to years in 20% of individuals (partial remission), and in others, full symptoms can persist for 2 or more years (chronic depression). Up to 10% of individuals with major depression will develop a manic episode (ie, bipolar I disorder [see below]). The suicide rate in patients with severe depression is 15%. Major depression often coexists with anxiety disorders, substance abuse disorders, and eating disorders.[13]

Pathophysiology

- Many neurochemical and structural abnormalities identified in HPA, HPT, and hypothalamic-growth hormone (GH) axes as well as in specific components of these systems (eg, ↑ CRF, ↑ cortisol)

- These neuroendocrine systems are controlled in part by norepinephrine, serotonin, acetylcholine (ACH), dopamine, and GABA; numerous abnormalities in neurotransmitter secretion and function are identified in depressed patients (see comprehensive reviews in references 94 and 95).

Presentation

Many depressed patients appear sad (tearful) and discouraged (brooding) and may claim to be "down in the dumps" or to lack interest in activities. Sadness may be denied initially but can be inferred from body language or facial expressions. Some depressed patients do not appear sad but are irritable, anxious, or apathetic. In primary care, somatic complaints are a common presentation in depressed patients.[96] Complaints that are more likely to indicate a diagnosis of depression include sleep disturbance, fatigue, nonspecific musculoskeletal complaints, back pain, motor tension, and shortness of breath. Patients with multiple complaints, vague complaints, or amplified complaints also are more likely to be depressed.[97] Depressive symptoms develop over days to weeks; some patients may experience a prodromal phase before full-blown symptoms appear.

Diagnosis/Screening Tools

Several reliable screening tools (patient self-reporting scales) such as the MINI Structured Interview (Parts A and C; see APPENDIX) can help identify persons likely to have depressive symptoms and prompt the clinician to conduct a diagnostic interview; many of these tools are useful in the primary care setting (Table 13).[90,96,98-100]

Table 13. Screening tools for depression in primary care[90,96,98]

- General Health Questionnaire (GHQ)
- Beck Depression Inventory (BDI)
- Geriatric Depression Scale (GDS)
- Goldberg Screen for Depressive Disorders
- Symptom-Driven Diagnostic System for Primary Care (SDDS-PC)
- Center for Epidemiologic Studies-Depression Scale (CES-D)
- Zung Self-Rating Depression Scale (ZSRDS)
- Inventory for Depressive Symptomatology (IDS)
- Primary Care Evaluation of Mental Disorders (PRIME-MD)
- Hamilton Rating Scale for Depression (HAM-D)

A careful and directed interview is needed to elicit symptoms of depression (Table 14), because patients with depression may have difficulty concentrating or remembering or may tend to deny or explain away certain symptoms. Also, somatic complaints may inadvertently steer the physician away from making a psychiatric diagnosis and toward ordering laboratory or other diagnostic tests. Because the presenting symptoms of many medical illnesses include sleep disturbance, fatigue, and nonspecific complaints, it may be useful to inquire about guilt, suicidality, or low self-esteem to aid in making a diagnosis.

Inquiry should be made into the patient's marital, occupational, or academic situation. A mental status exam should include information on suicidal thoughts.[90] The risk of suicide also can be assessed by asking a few short questions (Table 15). Physicians should not be reluctant to ask about suicide; many patients will speak directly about suicide, given an opportunity.[101]

Included in the *Diagnostic and Statistical Manual of Mental Disorders*, fourth edition (DSM-IV), are criteria for depressive subtypes such as psychotic (hallucinations, delusions), atypical, and melancholic. Some of the rating scales listed in Table 13 rate the severity of depressive symptoms and can be used to follow patients over time as a measure of improvement. Three DSM-IV mood disorders not discussed here (ie, premenstrual dysphoric disorder, minor depressive disorder, and recurrent brief depression) also may cause clinically, significantly impaired functioning and may require treatment.[13]

As many as one fourth of individuals with serious medical conditions (eg, diabetes, acquired immunodeficiency syndrome [AIDS], myocardial infarction [MI], cancer, stroke) develop depression.[102] Unfortunately, if this occurs, management of the medical condition becomes more complex and the prognosis of the depression less favorable.[13] Major depressive disorder must be differentiated from mood disorders caused by a medical condition (Table 16), substance abuse, or dementia (especially in the elderly).[90] No laboratory tests are diagnostic for major depressive disorder.

Table 14. Diagnostic criteria for major depressive disorder (adapted from reference 13, with permission). © Copyright 1994, American Psychiatric Association.

- ≥5 symptoms present nearly every day during a 2-week period; represents a change from previous functioning and causes clinically significant impairment in social or occupational functioning:
  - depressed mood most of the day (eg, feeling sad, empty, appearing tearful)[a]
  - markedly ↓ interest or pleasure in all or most activities most of the day[a]
  - significant (≥5%) ↑ or ↓ in weight or appetite when not dieting
  - insomnia or hypersomnia
  - psychomotor agitation or retardation
  - fatigue or loss of energy
  - feelings of worthlessness, excessive or inappropriate guilt
  - diminished ability to think or concentrate, indecisiveness
  - recurrent thoughts of death or suicide, suicide attempt or a specific plan for committing suicide
- Patient has never had a manic, hypomanic, or mixed episode

[a]≥1 of these symptoms needed to make the diagnosis.

Table 15. Questions to assess risk of suicide (adapted from reference 101, with permission). © Copyright 1997. Massachusetts Medical Society. All rights reserved.

- "Have you had thoughts about death or about killing yourself?"
  If yes, ask:
  - "Do you have a plan?"
  - "Are there means available (gun and bullets, poison)?"
  - "Have you actually rehearsed or practiced how you would kill yourself?"
  - "Do you tend to be impulsive?"
  - "Can you resist the impulse to do this?"
  - "Have you heard voices telling you to hurt or kill yourself?"
- Ask about previous attempts, especially the degree of intent
- Ask about suicide of family members

Referral

- Consider referral to a psychiatrist to clarify diagnosis, integrate pharmacologic treatment or deal with treatment refractoriness, initiate psychotherapy (to deal with life crises or difficulties), patient and family education, or electroconvulsive therapy (ECT)
- Consider referral to a psychologist or social worker for psychotherapy
- Psychiatric referral indicated for depression complicated by psychosis, suicidal intention, or past history of suicide attempts.

Table 16. Medical conditions associated with depressive symptoms (reproduced from reference 103, with permission)

System	Examples
Cardiovascular	Cardiomyopathy, cerebral ischemia, CHF, MI
Neurologic	Alzheimer's disease, multiple sclerosis, Parkinson's disease, head trauma, narcolepsy, brain tumors, Wilson's disease
Cancer	Pancreatic cancer, lung cancer
Endocrine	Hypothyroidism, hyperthyroidism, Cushing's disease, Addison's disease, hypoparathyroidism, hyperparathyroidism, hypoglycemia, pheochromocytoma, ovarian or testicular failure
Infectious diseases	Syphilis, mononucleosis, hepatitis, AIDS, tuberculosis, influenza, encephalitis, Lyme disease
Nutritional deficiencies	Folate, B_{12}, B_6, B_2, B_1, iron

Abbreviations defined in GLOSSARY.

Treatment

Treatment goals are to reduce and eliminate depressive signs and symptoms, restore the presymptomatic level of functioning, and reduce the likelihood of relapse. These goals often can be met with antidepressant drugs, psychotherapy, or the combination.[104]

Overview: Treatment of a depressive episode involves acute, continuation, and long-term (maintenance) phases. If a patient responds to acute treatment, continuation therapy is used to prevent relapse (return of symptoms within 6 months of the acute episode). Continuation therapy may be stopped if the patient is symptom free for 6 months or longer and is not at a high risk for recurrence. However, if new episodes develop months or years later (recurrence), maintenance therapy is needed to prevent further recurrence.[93,104] Treatment guidelines for major depression specifically developed for primary care physicians have been published by the Agency for Health Care Policy and Research (AHCPR)[104] (see RESOURCES for ordering information).

Antidepressant Selection: All antidepressants are equally effective, but side-effect profiles, dosing schedules, prior response, concurrent medical or psychiatric disorders (see Figure 6 and Table 17), drug interaction potential, and cost issues may make a particular antidepressant preferred for a specific patient.[93] Physician experience and patient preference also may guide drug selection. Regardless of the antidepressant chosen, full therapeutic doses must be used, and a full clinical response usually will not be evident before 4 to 6 weeks.[105] With appropriate treatment, approximately 70% of depressed patients can be expected to respond. In general, SSRIs are first-line therapy for acute, uncomplicated major depression because they are easy to use, better tolerated, and safer in overdose than TCAs. However, other newer agents with favorable side-effect profiles may also be first-line choices, including venlafaxine, nefazodone, and mirtazapine.

Comorbidity: Antidepressant selection is important if a concurrent medical condition is present (Table 17) because certain side effects may improve or exacerbate the underlying condition.[93] When two or more psychiatric disorders are present, physicians should focus on treatment of the one believed to be the primary or more serious condition, which also may lead to resolution of the other (Table 18).

Compliance with antidepressant therapy is a problem in as many as 90% of patients with mood disorders.[104] Primary care physicians can provide written and verbal education to patients, family members, or close acquaintances about the importance of adhering to the treatment regimen, the anticipated delay in response, and side effects.

Figure 6. Pharmacologic treatment approach to the patient with acute major depression (modified from reference 104; see also reference 106). Abbreviations defined in GLOSSARY.

EVALUATE and examine patient:
Assess suicide risk, presence of psychosis, melancholia

CONSIDER:
Concurrent medical or psychiatric disorders
Prior antidepressant response
Substance abuse

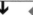

INITIATE pharmacologic therapy with SSRI, miscellaneous antidepressant (eg, bupropion, nefazodone, venlafaxine, mirtazapine), or TCA

ASSESS response at 1 or 2 weeks, monitor plasma level if TCA used, assess tolerability:

Full: Continue treatment 6 more weeks

Partial: Continue treatment, ↑ dose, monitor every 1 - 2 weeks

None: ↑ Dose and continue treatment for 1 more week. If in therapeutic plasma range and no response at 3 weeks, change to another antidepressant; monitor every 1 - 2 weeks

REASSESS response at 6 weeks:

Full (complete remission): Continue antidepressant at same dose for 4 - 9 months, then discontinue (taper over ≥4 weeks). Consider maintenance treatment in patients with ≥3 episodes

Partial or *None*: Change to another antidepressant
Consider psychiatric referral for augmentation or ECT

CONSIDER:
Psychiatric referral for difficult cases (ie, no response after one or two medication trials, deterioration, ↑ or new suicidal thoughts, frequent relapses, atypical symptoms, psychotic symptoms, manic symptoms, development of comorbid mental disorder, substance abuse)

Table 17. Antidepressant selection with comorbid medical disorders[93,102,103]

Condition	Prefer	Avoid
Cardiac disease (CAD, orthostatic hypotension, arrhythmias)	SSRIs, bupropion, mirtazapine	TCAs, MAOIs, trazodone (?)
Seizures, head trauma	SSRIs, MAOIs, desipramine, venlafaxine, mirtazapine	Maprotiline, clomipramine, bupropion, and other TCAs
Stroke	SSRIs, nortriptyline	
Dementia	SSRIs, trazodone, bupropion	Amitriptyline, clomipramine, protriptyline, amoxapine, and other TCAs
Parkinson's disease	SSRIs, amitriptyline, doxepin	Amoxapine, MAOIs
Asthma	SSRIs, nortriptyline	MAOIs (↑ risk of drug interactions)
Angle-closure glaucoma	SSRIs, bupropion, trazodone, nefazodone	Amitriptyline, clomipramine, protriptyline, amoxapine
Cancer	SSRIs, bupropion, mirtazapine, venlafaxine	TCAs, MAOIs

Abbreviations defined in GLOSSARY.

Table 18. Approach to the depressed patient with comorbid psychiatric disorders[106]

Comorbid disorder	Treatment approach
Substance dependence	Treat substance dependence first; if depression is still present, treat the depression
GAD	Treat depression first; anxiety usually resolves
Eating disorder or OCD	Treat eating disorder or OCD first; if depression is still present, treat the depression. Use agent effective in both eating disorder and major depression (eg, TCA, SSRI, or MAOI) or OCD and major depression (eg, SSRI or clomipramine)
PD	Treat PD first if it is of longer duration or has familial tendencies; otherwise, treat depression first. Use agent effective in both depression and PD (eg, SSRI or TCA)

Abbreviations defined in GLOSSARY.

ADOLESCENT DEPRESSION

Depression in adolescents can lead to declining academic performance, poor peer relationships, and family conflict. Suicide is one of the most feared consequences of adolescent depression. Therefore, timely diagnosis and treatment are important.[107]

Epidemiology

Depression occurs in approximately 5% of adolescents and is twice as common in girls as in boys.[108] Physicians who treat adults with depression should consider that children in the family may also have depression. Conversely, if a child with depression is being treated, the possibility of depression in a parent or sibling also should be considered. The high comorbidity of adolescent depression with anxiety disorders and substance abuse may increase the risk for suicide.[107] Predictors of suicidality in children and adolescents include preoccupation with themes of death, expressing suicidal thoughts, prior suicide attempts, and making "final arrangements," such as giving away prized possessions or making a will. Additional warning signs include sudden or extreme changes in sleeping patterns, eating habits, and school performance or behavior. Children who exhibit personality changes, such as unexplained nervousness, outbursts of anger, or apathy about appearance and health also may be at risk for suicide.

At least 50% of depressed adolescents will experience another episode within 3 years. Evidence suggests that adolescents with depression are at risk for developing adult depression; one third of adolescents with depressive symptoms may switch to mania.[108]

Presentation

Depressed adolescents have many of the same features of depression seen in adults (eg, dysphoric and worthless feelings, loss of interest in activities, low self-esteem, poor concentration, low energy level, and thoughts of death).[109] However, certain features of adolescent depression are unique, such as irritability. Depressed adolescents may complain about everything, are short tempered, and lose perspective. Parents may report that they are not getting along with the child, and the child reports that he or she is not getting along with friends. These children often have feelings of isolation because they feel that no one understands them or can help them.

Diagnosis/Screening Tools

Depressed adolescents take extreme measures to hide symptoms (eg, tearfulness, frequent crying) from friends, family members, and teachers. This diagnosis is sometimes missed because the adolescent does not outwardly appear depressed. Including a family member in the interview is helpful for clarification of external changes (appetite, sleep, school behavior).[108]

Treatment

Psychotherapy may help patients and their families become educated about the biologic basis of depression, and it may help young patients understand that the disease is not their fault.[108,110]

Pharmacologic treatment options in adolescent depression are similar to those in adults, although TCAs may be less effective.[108] The SSRIs are highly effective in children and adolescents and are well tolerated and safe, especially in overdose.[111] All agents in a class should be tried before changing to another class of antidepressant drug. Once an effective SSRI is identified, it should be continued in an appropriate dose for at least 1 year to prevent recurrences. The TCAs usually are reserved for SSRI treatment failure because several side effects (eg, sedation, weight gain, dry mouth, and constipation) are highly problematic for adolescents. Serious cardiac side effects including sudden death have been reported in children receiving TCAs.

DEPRESSION IN THE ELDERLY

Depression in community-dwelling elderly persons is a major public health problem that often is underdiagnosed and undertreated. Its symptom profile may appear to be related to the normal aging process or to concomitant medical illnesses.[103,112]

Epidemiology

Major depression, according to DSM-IV criteria, is uncommon (1% or 2%) in elderly persons, but a high proportion of older individuals (up to 20%) have subthreshold symptoms of depression that cause functional disability and suffering.[89,112] An even higher proportion (up to 40%) of hospitalized or nursing-home-based elderly patients exhibit some form of depression.[113]

Presentation

Symptoms of depression in the elderly have an insidious onset, are less prominent than in younger persons, and may be mistaken for signs of normal aging or for a comorbid medical illness. Elderly persons may complain of changes in sleep, loss of appetite or weight loss, apathy, anergia, or social withdrawal. Depressive symptoms in elderly persons may increase their risk for a subsequent decline in physical function.[114] Also, physicians should be aware of the high rates of suicide in untreated depressed elderly, especially Caucasian males.[112]

Treatment

Once recognized, depression in the elderly is a treatable disorder, as treatable as in younger patients. Antidepressants are just as effective as in younger persons, but risks of adverse drug reactions may be greater (see DRUG USE IN THE ELDERLY, page 165). Drug interactions may be more likely because the elderly usually are taking multiple medications.

Among the TCAs, nortriptyline or desipramine is preferred because these two agents cause less orthostatic hypotension and fewer adverse effects. The

SSRIs also are highly effective in the elderly, are well tolerated, and show long-term efficacy.[115] Bupropion is effective and well tolerated but may cause activation. Nefazodone and trazodone have sedative effects that can be useful if the patient is agitated, but these drugs also cause significant orthostatic hypotension. MAOIs or ECT can be effective, the latter especially so in severely depressed or delusional patients. In any case, use of low doses of antidepressants, increased gradually, and maintainence treatment for an appropriate duration to avoid relapse should be the approach to treatment.

DYSTHYMIC DISORDER

Dysthymic disorder is the chronic presence (ie, lasting ≥2 years) of depressed mood for more days than not with other depressive symptoms that do not meet criteria for major depression. It is distinct from major depression, but major depression often occurs in patients with dysthymia, so-called double depression.

Epidemiology

The lifetime prevalence of dysthymic disorder has been estimated to be 6.4%[3]; it is at least twice as common in women as in men. Dysthymic disorder is chronic and often progresses to major depression. It also is associated with a high degree of functional disability, exceeded only by congestive heart failure (CHF).[116] Dysthymia is more common in first-degree relatives of patients diagnosed with major depression than in the general population, and it frequently coexists with personality, anxiety, and substance abuse disorders.[13]

Pathophysiology

- Cause(s) not as well defined as other mood disorders
- Likely shares a pathophysiology similar to that of major depression.

Presentation

In patients with dysthymic disorder, generalized feelings of inadequacy, loss of interest, social withdrawal, guilty feelings, or decreased productivity are more common than vegetative symptoms relating to sleeping or eating.[13] Many patients state, "I've always been this way," or feel that they are just always "down in the dumps."

Diagnosis/Screening Tools

Making a diagnosis of dysthymia (Table 19) can be difficult because the symptoms are similar to those of depression but differ in duration (greater) and severity (milder).[89] Whereas depression is episodic and can usually be differentiated from a normal baseline status, dysthymia is unremitting and may be perceived as the baseline status.[116] Direct questioning is needed to elicit symptoms because dysthymic patients may believe their mood to be part of their personality. The MINI (Part B; see APPENDIX) may be a useful tool in the primary care setting.

Table 19. Diagnostic criteria for dysthymic disorder (adapted from reference 13, with permission). © Copyright 1994, American Psychiatric Association.

Depressed mood most of the day, more days than not, for ≥2 years

- While depressed, patient has ≥2 symptoms:
  - ↓ appetite or overeating
  - insomnia or hypersomnia
  - low energy or fatigue
  - low self-esteem
  - poor concentration or difficulty making decisions
  - feelings of hopelessness
- During the 2-year period:
  - person has never been without the symptoms for >2 months at a time
  - major depressive disorder has not been present
  - manic, mixed, or hypomanic episodes have not been present
- Symptoms not due to medications, substances of abuse, or a medical condition (eg, hypothyroidism)
- Clinically significant distress or impairment in social, occupational, or other important areas of functioning

Referral

- Although recent data advocate pharmacotherapy for first-line treatment, psychotherapy also may be needed for complete recovery.

Treatment

Dysthymic disorder often responds to SSRIs or TCAs, but a response may not be evident for 2 or 3 months.[116] Treatment guidelines (as outlined in the section on MAJOR DEPRESSIVE DISORDER; see page 26) should be followed. Because of the chronic nature of dysthymic disorder, long-term maintenance therapy (≥1 year) will help sustain the benefits of acute treatment.

BIPOLAR DISORDER

Bipolar disorder involves periods of mania or hypomania often alternating with depression (Table 20). Bipolar disorder frequently appears at a relatively early age and thus can significantly and adversely impact school attendance, ability to train for and hold a job, and development of social and personal relationships.

Table 20. Differentiating features of bipolar disorder

Type	Features
Bipolar I	≥1 manic or mixed episode, usually with major depressive episodes
Bipolar II	≥1 hypomanic episode with ≥1 major depressive episode; no manic episodes
Mixed or dysphoric	Manic and depressive symptoms occur simultaneously
Rapid cycling	≥4 episodes of mood disturbance in previous 12 months

Epidemiology

Approximately 1.3% of US adults have bipolar disorder. The onset of bipolar disorder usually begins between the ages of 15 and 19, but treatment may not begin until several years later. Unlike major depression, bipolar I disorder is equally common in males and females[3] and is common in first-degree relatives of affected individuals. Bipolar II disorder is less common than bipolar I disorder, more common in women, and possibly more common in the postpartum period. Bipolar disorder is a chronic, recurrent, and episodic condition. Most patients (80%) having one manic episode will have another; the episodes become progressively more severe and less responsive to treatment in many, if not most, patients. For many patients, the cycle length shortens with each successive episode and stabilizes at one or two episodes per year. A typical untreated bipolar patient will experience 10 or more episodes during his or her lifetime.[117] Suicide attempts occur in approximately 25% of patients with bipolar I disorder, with 15% of patients completing such attempts.[13]

Pathophysiology

- Abnormalities in neuroendocrine (eg, HPA, HPT), neurotransmitter (eg, norepinephrine, serotonin, dopamine, GABA, ACH), and second-messenger systems and brain-imaging studies.[94]

Presentation

A first bipolar episode can be either manic (usually in men) or depressive (usually in women); several years may pass until the next episode.[117] Patients in a depressive phase (ie, bipolar depression) display typical features (as described in the section on MAJOR DEPRESSIVE DISORDER; see page 23), although some symptoms (hypersomnia, psychomotor retardation) may be more common in bipolar depression. However, the duration of bipolar depressive episodes tends to be shorter than those of unipolar depression but longer than manic or hypomanic episodes.

The typical presentation of the manic phase is elevated mood, but mixed features (Table 20) occur in a substantial percentage of patients. Although this quality may seem euphoric and happily contagious, family members or close acquaintances recognize it as excessive or irritating.[13] A manic patient may go without sleep for days but not be tired; speech often is loud, rapid, and theatrical. Clothing and makeup suddenly are out of character (eg, dressing in a provocative way).

Manic patients often do not recognize that they are ill and thus resist attempts to be treated. Additional characteristics are described in the diagnostic criteria below (Table 21).[13]

Diagnosis/Screening Tools

There are many diagnostic subtypes for bipolar disorder in which patients can be classified based on the most recent episode or by certain presenting features; refer to DSM-IV for additional information on these subtypes.[13] There are no diagnostic laboratory tests for bipolar disorder. The MINI (Part D; see APPENDIX) may be useful in identifying episodes of mania or hypomania.

Mania needs to be differentiated from schizophrenia and from mood disorders caused by general medical conditions (eg, Parkinson's disease, stroke, thyroid disorders, autoimmune conditions, viral infections, and certain cancers).[13] Mania occurring in someone older than 40 or 50 years may be caused by a medical condition or the effects of one or another medication. Hypomanic episodes may be confused with the period of euthymia that normally follows remission of a major depressive episode. Substance abuse must be ruled out. Individuals with bipolar II disorder often do not recall periods of hypomania; information needs to be obtained from family or other outside sources.[117]

Referral

- Refer patients with suspected bipolar disorder for prompt psychiatric evaluation

- Immediately transfer anyone with severe mania or depression who is deemed to be at risk for self-harm or harm to others to an inpatient facility

- Refer stabilized patients and their family members to providers skilled in group or individual counseling for education about medication compliance (eg, serum-level monitoring, dietary/fluid issues with lithium [see page 106]), substance abuse awareness, maintaining regular sleep habits, and stress management.

Table 21. Broad diagnostic criteria for bipolar disorder (adapted from reference 13, with permission). © Copyright 1994, American Psychiatric Association.

Type	Diagnostic criteria
Bipolar I	• One manic episode (distinct period of abnormally and persistently elevated, expansive, or irritable mood, lasting ≥1 week) • Usually with major depressive episode[a] • Manic episode causes marked impairment in occupational functioning or in social or personal activities, or is severe enough to require hospitalization, or psychotic features are present
Bipolar II	• One major depressive episode[a] • One hypomanic episode (distinct period of persistently elevated, expansive, or irritable mood lasting ≥4 days) • No manic episodes • Delusions or hallucinations are not present and the severity does not necessitate hospitalization • Symptoms cause clinically significant (but not marked) distress or impairment in social or occupational functioning
Bipolar I and Bipolar II (mixed)	• Three significant symptoms (≥4 if mood only irritable) present during the period of mood disturbance: – ↑ self-esteem or grandiosity – ↓ need for sleep – more talkative than usual or pressure to keep talking – flight of ideas, subjective feeling of racing thoughts – distractibility toward unimportant or irrelevant stimuli – ↑ in goal-directed activity or psychomotor agitation – excessive involvement in pleasurable activities that have ↑ potential for painful consequences (eg, sexual indiscretion, unrestrained buying sprees, foolish investments)

[a]See Table 14.

Treatment

The primary treatment goal is to reduce morbidity and mortality by reducing the frequency and severity of episodes and by stabilizing mood between episodes.[117] Acute management is determined by whether the patient is in a manic or depressive phase. Much more is known about the treatment of mania than about bipolar depression, for which the treatment approach has largely been extrapolated from that of unipolar depression.[117-119]

Treatment noncompliance in bipolar patients is common for four reasons. First, manic patients often deny their illness and see no need for treatment. Second, many patients (especially during hypomania) enjoy the extra energy and feelings that are present during manic phases. Third, the medication regimen for many bipolar patients is extraordinarily complicated, with multiple daily dosing of one or more drugs. It is not unusual for bipolar patients to be treated with two or three mood stabilizers and an antidepressant. Finally, medication side effects may be unacceptable or intolerable for some patients. Primary care physicians can promote compliance with treatment and reinforce the need for stress management and good sleep habits to reduce the risk of precipitating a manic cycle.

Acute Mania: Lithium and valproic acid are the drugs of choice for acute management of classic, euphoric mania (Figure 7). About 80% of persons will show some response to lithium within 2 weeks. Carbamazepine or valproic acid may be of special value in mixed or rapid-cycling bipolar disorder (≥4 episodes/y) and also when lithium is not tolerated or is ineffective. Antipsychotics or benzodiazepines can provide rapid stabilization of mood during the first week of lithium treatment. Treatment-resistant mania requires a multidrug regimen, addition of an atypical antipsychotic (eg, clozapine, olanzapine, quetiapine, risperidone), or ECT.[117,119] Potentially useful adjuncts to current mood-stabilizing therapy in acute mania include some calcium channel blockers, thyroid hormone in rapid cyclers, and newer anticonvulsants (eg, gabapentin, lamotrigine).[120]

Acute Bipolar Depression: Mood-stabilizing therapy (eg, lithium, valproic acid, carbamazepine) is typically required in addition to antidepressant therapy for acute bipolar I depression (Figure 8); it sometimes is omitted in bipolar II depression or mild depression. Although mood stabilizers may have acute antidepressant effects and may be effective as monotherapy,[121-123] most bipolar patients require an antidepressant such as an SSRI or bupropion.[124] The SSRIs are well tolerated and may be associated with a lower frequency of switching into mania (see page 40). The TCAs probably should be avoided because of their lethality in overdose situations (suicide attempts). A response to antidepressant therapy may take up to 6 or 8 weeks. Adjunctive benzodiazepine therapy for insomnia may be needed. The management of patients with treatment-resistant bipolar depression is complex. Changing to another antidepressant (eg, MAOI) may be helpful; ECT is also useful, especially in psychotic bipolar depression.[117,119,121] However, these patients often are a suicide risk and probably should be referred to a psychiatrist.

Figure 7. Pharmacologic treatment approach to the patient with acute mania.[117,119] Abbreviations defined in GLOSSARY.

EVALUATE and examine patient:
Features of episode (ie, classic [euphoric], mixed, rapid cycling)
Presence of psychosis, agitation, insomnia
Patient safety, risk of harm to self
Ability to be treated in an outpatient setting (compliance, family support)

CONSIDER:
Previous treatment response
Concurrent drug therapy or substance abuse (interaction potential)
Concurrent medical conditions (eg, renal or hepatic disease)

INITIATE mood-stabilizing therapy:
- Classic mania: lithium or valproic acid
- Mixed: valproic acid, lithium, or carbamazepine
- Rapid cycling: valproic acid or carbamazepine

Monitor serum levels: ↑ as tolerated and as serum levels dictate. Avoid lithium in renal disease, avoid anticonvulsant mood stabilizers in hepatic disease

INITIATE adjunctive therapy if needed:
- Psychotic features: antipsychotic
- Agitation or insomnia: benzodiazepine

ASSESS response:
Lithium: monitor serum levels at least twice weekly until stable, then weekly. Monitor baseline renal function, electrolytes, hematologic parameters. Response delayed 1 - 2 weeks
Anticonvulsant mood stabilizers: monitor serum levels as needed

CONSIDER:
- Immediate psychiatric referral for severe symptoms, suicidal, or psychotic features
- Psychiatric referral if no response or incomplete response after 1 - 3 weeks, or if symptoms worsen or new features develop suddenly
- Maintenance mood-stabilizing therapy with lithium or valproic acid
(bipolar I: after two manic episodes or one severe episode or strong family history; bipolar II: after three hypomanic episodes)

Figure 8. Pharmacologic treatment approach to the patient with acute bipolar depression.[117,119] Abbreviations defined in GLOSSARY.

EVALUATE and examine patient:
Severity of episode
Presence of psychosis, insomnia
Patient safety, risk of harm to self, others

CONSIDER:
Previous treatment response, rapid cycling?
Concurrent drug therapy or substance abuse (interaction potential)
Concurrent medical conditions

INITIATE mood-stabilizing therapy (see Figure 7):
- Mild to moderate symptoms: add antidepressant (eg, SSRI or bupropion)
- Severe symptoms: add antidepressant (eg, SSRI or bupropion)
- Psychotic symptoms: add antidepressant plus atypical antipsychotic or ECT
- Avoid TCAs in patients considered rapid cyclers

INITIATE adjunctive therapy if needed:
Benzodiazepine for insomnia or use sedating antidepressant

ASSESS response after several days:
Monitor mood-stabilizing therapy (see Figure 7)
Maintenance mood-stabilizing therapy with lithium or valproic acid
(bipolar I: after two manic episodes or one severe episode or strong family history; bipolar II: after three hypomanic episodes)

CONSIDER:
- Immediate psychiatric referral or hospitalization for severely depressed, suicidal, or psychotic patients with bipolar depression
- Psychiatric referral if no response or incomplete response after 1 - 3 weeks, or if symptoms worsen or new features develop suddenly
- Referral for education, group therapy, family counseling, psychotherapy

A controversial topic in the treatment of bipolar depression is whether antidepressants cause mania or reduce the cycle length.[125,126] It is clear that TCAs may cause between 30% and 70% of bipolar depressed patients to switch into mania or hypomania,[121] but that does not necessarily mean they change overt cycle length or frequency. Whether all antidepressants pose a risk or whether some pose less of a risk is not known because this issue has not been systematically evaluated in placebo-controlled trials and because untreated bipolar depressed patients have an inherently greater risk of switching to mania. SSRIs, MAOIs, or bupropion may have a lower switch risk or may cause a milder or shorter manic episode,[121,127] but this has not been shown conclusively. In patients with a history of rapid cycling, the lowest effective antidepressant dose should be used for the shortest possible time.

Continuation and Maintenance Therapy: Once the acute depressive episode has stabilized, mood-stabilizing therapy is continued to prevent cycling to the opposite pole; antidepressant therapy is tapered gradually. Maintenance mood-stabilizing therapy (possibly lifelong) is then used to prevent occurrence of new episodes.[117,119] Maintenance lithium reduces the frequency and severity of both mania and bipolar depression and stabilizes mood between cycles; it also reduces the risk of mortality.[122] Emerging data suggest that valproic acid is effective for maintenance therapy and may be better tolerated than lithium.[117,119,128] Some atypical antipsychotics (eg, olanzapine, risperidone, quetiapine, clozapine) may provide mood stabilization but have not yet been studied under controlled conditions.

Insomnia

Among all sleep disorders, the most common presentation to the primary care physician is primary insomnia. Insomnia and residual daytime sleepiness have an important impact on a patient's health and occupational and social performance. Persons with insomnia also may be at greater risk for serious accidents.[129] Although effective interventions are available, if not properly diagnosed, short-term insomnia can lead to chronic insomnia, which is much less amenable to treatment. Other primary sleep disorders, including hypersomnia (excessive sleepiness for >1 mo), narcolepsy (irresistible sleep attacks), or circadian rhythm sleep disorders (caused by jet lag, shift work), are not discussed in this handbook.

Epidemiology

In the general population, the 1-year prevalence rate of complaints of insomnia is 30% to 40%; in sleep disorder clinics, approximately 15% to 25% of patients with complaints of insomnia are diagnosed with primary insomnia.[13] The disorder is more common in women, and the prevalence rate increases with age;[130] primary insomnia is rare before early adulthood. Difficulty falling asleep is a more common complaint in younger adults, whereas early-morning awakening or intermittent nighttime wakening is more common in older adults. The course of primary insomnia is variable; it often develops suddenly during times of stress but may continue long after the acute stressor has resolved.

Pathophysiology

- Acute symptoms usually caused by psychological stress related to life events, travel (crossing time zones, sleeping in unfamiliar environments), poor sleep hygiene, or conditioned anxiety to bed/sleeping.[130]

Presentation

Patients with primary insomnia report a great deal of difficulty falling asleep and intermittent waking. They also may complain of restless or poor-quality (nonrestorative) sleep. Patients may feel irritable during the daytime and report decreased energy and concentration.[13] The patient's preoccupation and frustration with his or her inability to sleep perpetuates the sleep disorder cycle. Sleep hygiene often is very poor in patients with insomnia. For example, the patient will lie in a bed in which he or she has been unable to sleep, get frustrated or anxious, and therefore become negatively conditioned not to sleep in that bed. Chronic primary insomnia may be a risk factor for or an early symptom of mood or anxiety disorders.[130] Inappropriate use of alcohol or hypnotic drugs to promote sleep or stimulants or caffeine to maintain daytime alertness may progress to a substance abuse disorder.

Diagnosis/Screening Tools

A diagnosis of primary insomnia is made when a patient reports difficulty getting to sleep, difficulty maintaining sleep, or nonrestorative sleep for 1 month or more (Table 22).[13]

Table 22. Diagnostic criteria for primary insomnia (adapted from reference 13, with permission). © Copyright 1994, American Psychiatric Association.

- ≥1 month's duration of difficulty getting to sleep or maintaining sleep, or nonrestorative (unrefreshing) sleep
- Clinically significant distress or impairment in social, occupational, or other functioning
- Does not occur in relation to another primary sleep disorder, during the course of a mental disorder (eg, depression) or general medical condition, or substance/medication use

Early-morning awakening may indicate depression, difficulty in falling asleep may point to an anxiety disorder, and early-morning awakening with respiratory distress or a sense of dread may indicate PD.[131] Important information can be obtained from household members or bed partners with regard to snoring or behavior during sleep (eg, nightmares, apnea, restless leg syndrome, etc). Coexisting mood or anxiety disorders, medical conditions, or substance abuse (eg, alcohol, caffeine, nicotine) must be ruled out as causes of insomnia symptoms.

Having the patient complete a sleep log for 2 weeks may be useful in defining the exact symptoms and pattern of sleep. Entries might include information about mealtimes, bedtime, time and number of awakenings, use of alcohol, medications (Table 23), exercise, and duration of sleep.[130]

Table 23. Medications that may cause insomnia[130]

Drug class	Common examples
Anticholinergics	Ipratropium bromide
Antihypertensives	β-Blockers, clonidine, methyldopa, reserpine
Antineoplastics	Daunorubicin, goserelin acetate, interferon α, leuprolide acetate, medroxyprogesterone, pentostatin
CNS stimulants	Methylphenidate
Hormones	Cortisone, oral contraceptives, progesterone, thyroid preparations
Sympathomimetic amines	Bronchodilators, decongestants, theophylline
Miscellaneous	Caffeine[a], levodopa, nicotine, phenytoin, quinidine

Abbreviations defined in GLOSSARY.
[a]Often included in OTC analgesics or cough-cold preparations.

Other than sleep laboratory abnormalities (see reference 13), there are no definitive laboratory or physical findings to aid in diagnosing primary insomnia. However, patients may have a fatigued appearance and may have stress-related tension headaches, dyspepsia, or muscle tension.[13]

Referral

- Refer patients with chronic insomnia symptoms not helped by short-term drug therapy, excessive daytime sleepiness, sleep-related cardiorespiratory problems, or abnormal sleep behavior to a sleep medicine specialist.[131]

Treatment

A combination of educational and behavioral intervention often supplemented with short-term pharmacologic management (Table 24) is used to treat primary insomnia.[130,132] Although hypnotic drugs are more effective acutely, behavioral changes related to sleep hygiene are needed to sustain good sleep habits over the long term. Few data support long-term use of benzodiazepines in chronic insomnia.

Table 24. Drug treatment principles for primary insomnia[130]

- Use the lowest effective dose
- Dose intermittently (two or four times/wk)
- Encourage short-term use (≤4 wk)
- Gradually discontinue therapy
- Monitor for rebound insomnia

Hypnotic agents commonly used for short-term management of insomnia include benzodiazepines and zolpidem; nonbarbiturate hypnotics (eg, chloral hydrate) are used less often. Product selection is based on the pattern of symptoms and patient features. Use of hypnotics should be avoided in patients with restrictive chest disease (ie, due to morbid obesity) or obstructive sleep apnea.[131]

Benzodiazepines and Zolpidem: Benzodiazepines with long half-lives ($t_{1/2}$) (eg, flurazepam, quazepam) may reduce nighttime awakenings or daytime anxiety, but residual daytime sleepiness (hangover) could be a problem, especially in the elderly, who are prone to falls.[133] Longer-acting agents are less likely to be associated with rebound insomnia with prolonged use. Short- or intermediate-acting agents with inactive metabolites (eg, temazepam [see Table 68], zolpidem) promote rapid sleep onset. They are not usually associated with daytime sleepiness but may cause rebound insomnia when therapy is stopped.[130,131] Zolpidem (see page 128) may be better tolerated than benzodiazepines. Over-the-counter (OTC) sleep products (ie, antihistamines such as diphenhydramine [Nytol, Sominex]) are not consistently effective and may impair the quality of sleep as well as the next day's performance.[130] They also may cause confusion in elderly patients.

Antidepressants: Sedating TCAs (eg, trimipramine, amitriptyline), doxepin (see Table 41), and trazodone have gained popularity for the short-term management of insomnia, although there is little controlled evidence of their efficacy. These agents are associated with anticholinergic side effects, orthostatic hypotension, and possible effects on cardiac conduction, and are dangerous in overdose.

Somatization Disorder

The general category of somatoform disorders includes conditions such as somatization disorder highlighted by chronic, recurring physical symptoms that suggest or mimic a medical condition and that are not fully explained by a medical diagnosis, substance abuse, or other mental disorder. In the community, actual somatization disorder that fulfills DSM-IV criteria[13] is relatively rare, but somatic manifestations of other disorders (eg, depression, PD, anxiety) are very common[134-136] (also see MAJOR DEPRESSIVE DISORDER, page 22, PANIC DISORDER, page 3). Not unexpectedly, somatoform disorders are costly in terms of physician time, frustration, and healthcare expenses related to specialist referral; unnecessary diagnostic and laboratory tests; and inappropriate drug or surgical treatment.[96,137,138]

Epidemiology

Lifetime prevalence rates for somatization disorder range from 0.2% to 2%; in the US, it occurs almost exclusively in women. Symptoms often develop in adolescence and full diagnostic criteria usually are met by age 25. About one fourth of female first-degree relatives of a woman with somatization disorder will develop the condition. Male relatives have a higher risk of substance-related disorders or personality disorders.[13]

Pathophysiology

- Complex; unclear why some patients express psychologic distress as physical symptoms.[137]

Presentation

Patients with somatization disorder have multiple and continual pain, and GI, sexual, or pseudoneurologic complaints. Menstrual problems are one early symptom in women. After many extensive workups, few to no physical findings are found to support the complaints. Commonly, patients see several physicians simultaneously for treatment of their various complaints; therefore, a thorough drug history is needed to avoid potentially serious drug interactions.

Diagnosis/Screening Tools

Somatic complaints are common in patients with depression.[96] However, a somatic presentation of depression differs from actual somatization disorder (Table 25). Somatization disorder is suggested with physical complaints that involve multiple organ systems, that began at an early age, and that are without physical signs or structural or laboratory abnormalities. There are no diagnostic laboratory tests for somatization disorder.

Table 25. Diagnostic criteria for somatization disorder (adapted from reference 13, with permission). © Copyright 1994, American Psychiatric Association.

- Multiple physical complaints beginning before age 30, occurring over several years, and resulting in treatment being sought or significant impairment of social or occupational functioning
- *All* of the following:
  - ≥4 different pain symptoms (eg, head, abdomen, back, joints, extremities, chest, rectum, or during menstruation, urination, or sexual intercourse)
  - ≥2 GI symptoms (eg, nausea, bloating, vomiting other than during pregnancy, diarrhea, or multiple food intolerance)
  - 1 sexual symptom other than pain (eg, sexual indifference, erectile or ejaculatory dysfunction, irregular menses, ↑ menstrual bleeding, vomiting during pregnancy)
  - 1 pseudoneurologic symptom not limited to pain (eg, impaired balance or coordination, paralysis, difficulty swallowing, aphonia, urinary retention, hallucinations, loss of touch or pain sensation, double vision, blindness, deafness, amnesia, etc)
- Symptoms not fully explained by a known medical condition, effects of a medication, or drug of abuse or, if a medical condition is present, the complaints or resulting social or occupational dysfunction are greater than expected
- Symptoms are not intentionally produced or feigned

Abbreviations defined in GLOSSARY.

Because the list of diagnostic criteria for somatization disorder is long, a modified list of seven common symptoms may identify (80% likelihood) patients with this disorder[139] (Table 26).

Table 26. Seven-symptom screening test for somatization disorder[139]

- Shortness of breath
- Painful extremities
- Amnesia
- Burning sensation in sex organs
- Dysmenorrhea
- Lump in throat
- Vomiting

Referral

- Avoid multiple medical specialist referrals
- Reserve formal psychiatric consultation/referral for complicated or severe cases.

Treatment

No pharmacologic treatment for somatization disorder has been demonstrated to be effective, although some patients may respond to SSRIs. The primary treatment approach is psychotherapeutic. Chronic illness is a way of life for these patients, and medical treatment for physical complaints is not typically indicated. General principles to guide primary care physicians are shown below (Table 27); these interventions may reduce overall healthcare expenditures associated with this disorder.[137,140]

Table 27. Treatment principles for somatization disorder[137,140]

- Encourage use of one primary care physician; avoid multiple specialist referrals
- Develop a sound doctor-patient relationship
- Use straightforward predominantly psychologic interventions
- Avoid unnecessary diagnostic procedures, drugs, or surgeries
- Offer regularly scheduled, brief visits every 4 - 6 weeks, including a brief physical exam
- Avoid "as-needed" visits

Substance Use Disorders

Substance use disorders comprise both abuse and dependence. Only four of 11 common substances (eg, cocaine, alcohol, opiates, and nicotine) are reviewed herein, but two (ie, cocaine and alcohol) share diagnostic features with other commonly abused substances (ie, amphetamines and sedative-hypnotics/anxiolytics, respectively). Core symptoms of abuse and dependence are similar regardless of the substance being abused. Thus, in DSM-IV, general diagnostic criteria are provided (Tables 28 and 29). Issues specific to alcohol, cocaine, and opiates are included in the appropriate sections.

Table 28. Diagnostic criteria for general substance abuse disorder (adapted from reference 13, with permission). © Copyright 1994, American Psychiatric Association.

Maladaptive pattern of recurrent substance use leading to clinically significant impairment or distress, with ≥1 of the following occurring within a 12-month period:

- Failure to fulfill major role obligations at work, school, or home
- Substance use in physically hazardous situations (eg, driving a car)
- Recurrent substance-related legal problems
- Continued use despite persistent or recurrent social or interpersonal problems caused by or exacerbated by the effects of the substance (eg, arguments with spouse about intoxication)

Table 29. Diagnostic criteria for substance dependence disorder (adapted from reference 13, with permission). © Copyright 1994, American Psychiatric Association.

Maladaptive pattern of substance use causing clinically significant impairment or distress, and ≥3 of the following occurring within a 12-month period:

- Tolerance (↑ amount of substance needed to achieve intoxication, desired effect, or marked ↓ effect with continued use of same amount)
- Withdrawal (characteristic withdrawal syndrome for the substance, or the same or closely related substance is taken to relieve or avoid withdrawal symptoms)
- Substance often taken in ↑ amounts or over a longer period than intended
- Persistent desire or unsuccessful efforts to ↓ or control use
- ↑ Time spent in activities to obtain or use the substance or recover from its effects
- Important social, occupational, or recreational activities given up or reduced because of substance use
- Use continued despite knowledge of having persistent or recurrent physical or psychological problems likely to have been caused or exacerbated by the substance

ALCOHOL ABUSE AND DEPENDENCE

Alcoholism is a huge public health problem associated with tremendous loss of life due to accidents, suicide, violence, and alcohol-related illness. Primary care physicians have an important role in the early detection and treatment of alcohol-related problems,[141] especially in the elderly, in whom such problems often go unrecognized.[142]

Epidemiology

Alcohol dependence is common in the US, eclipsed in frequency only by major depression. Lifetime prevalence rates of alcohol abuse and dependence range from 14%[143] to 23.5%,[3] and use and dependence may be up to five times more common in males, although rates are rising in the female population. Most individuals who develop alcohol-related disorders do so by their late 30s. In severe alcohol withdrawal, the risk of mortality is about 5%.[144] Alcohol abuse and dependence frequently coexist with other mental disorders;[145] poly-substance abuse also is common because alcohol may be used as a substitute for or to alleviate undesirable symptoms associated with abuse or dependence of other substances.[13] Alcohol abuse is common in bipolar I and bipolar II disorders, with lifetime prevalences of approximately 50% and 60%, respectively.

Pathophysiology

- Alcohol craving and consumption may be linked to dysfunction of several neurotransmitter systems (eg, serotonin, dopamine, GABA)
- Alcohol may ↑ endogenous opioid activity
- Alcohol dependence may be partly due to genetic factors.[146]

Presentation

Persons who are acutely intoxicated with alcohol have slurred speech; unsteady gait; tremor; impaired judgment, attention, or memory; nystagmus; and possibly, stupor. In severe cases, amnesia (blackout) is present.

Persons in alcohol withdrawal can have mild symptoms (nausea, headache, irritability) or severe symptoms (tachycardia, perspiration, tremu-lousness, seizures). Delirium tremens (confusion, severe agitation, hallucina-tions) may appear several days after initial withdrawal symptoms.[147] Persons who are malnourished or otherwise compromised (eg, electrolyte imbalance, infection) may be at greater risk for cardiovascular collapse.[13,144]

Diagnosis/Screening Tools

There are no specific diagnostic criteria for either alcohol abuse or dependence other than the general criteria provided in Tables 28 and 29. Evidence for acute alcohol use can be obtained by measurement of alcohol in blood, breath, or urine. Physical findings in chronic alcohol users include gastritis or ulcers, cirrhosis, pancreatitis, mild hypertension, hepatomegaly, peripheral neuropathies, cardiomyopathies, and cognitive defects due to vita-min (especially thiamine) deficiencies. These alcohol-related problems are especially common in the elderly.[142] A fairly sensitive laboratory marker of acute heavy drinking is elevated γ-glutamyltransferase (GGT) activity (>30 units). However, normal GGT levels do not rule out heavy episodic drinking during 2 weeks prior to evaluation. Other chronic laboratory changes in heavy drinkers include elevations in mean corpuscular volume (MCV), liver function tests (LFTs), blood lipids, and uric acid.[13]

The CAGE questionnaire (Table 30) is a useful, brief screening tool; an affirmative answer to two or more questions is highly specific and sensitive for alcoholism.[147,148] Other tools, such as the MINI (Part J; see APPENDIX), the Michigan Alcoholism Screening Test (MAST; score >5 indicates alcoholism),[149] or Alcohol Use Disorders Identification Test (AUDIT), also may be helpful.[142,150] Laboratory tests are not appropriate for screening.[151]

Table 30. The CAGE questionnaire[147,148]

Have you ever:
- **C**: felt you should **C**ut down on your drinking?
- **A**: been **A**nnoyed at others for criticizing your drinking?
- **G**: felt bad or **G**uilty about your drinking?
- **E**: taken a drink first thing in the morning (**E**ye opener) to get rid of a hangover or steady your nerves?

An affirmative answer to ≥2 questions is highly specific and sensitive for alcoholism.

Referral
- Refer patients to self-help groups (eg, Alcoholics Anonymous) or inpatient or outpatient rehabilitation programs
- Hospitalize persons with severe symptoms or other medical problems (eg, malnutrition, infection).

Treatment
Primary care physicians have a significant role in reducing excessive alcohol use through screening, early intervention, counseling, and education.[141] Pharmacotherapy alone has no role in the management of alcohol abuse or dependence but acts as an adjunct to psychotherapy or self-help programs. Drug treatment may involve benzodiazepines (for prevention or treatment of mild to moderate withdrawal symptoms), disulfiram (which renders alcohol intake an aversive experience), or naltrexone (an anticraving agent).[152] Antidepressants may be indicated if clinical depression is present after 1 to 3 weeks.

Benzodiazepines: Like alcohol, benzodiazepines enhance GABA-ergic transmission and thus are useful for outpatient management of mild or moderate alcohol withdrawal symptoms. A typical regimen involves using a long-acting benzodiazepine (eg, diazepam 10 mg every 6 h) to control withdrawal symptoms, and then increasing or decreasing the dose as needed for lack of control or excess sedation, respectively. Intermediate-acting agents without active metabolites (eg, lorazepam, alprazolam) may be used if hepatic function is impaired. In either case, the dose is gradually tapered during the next week and then stopped. See BENZODIAZEPINES (page 113) for specific information on safety, drug interactions, etc.

Disulfiram: Disulfiram (Antabuse®) is approved as an adjunct to nonpharmacologic treatments of alcohol dependence. By inhibiting aldehyde dehydrogenase, the enzyme responsible for the oxidation of aldehyde (ethanol), blood levels of acetaldehyde increase and cause facial flushing, throbbing headache, tachycardia, hypotension, nausea, and vomiting. The initial dose is 500 mg once daily (QD) for 1 or 2 weeks; the usual maintenance dose is 250 mg QD. Disulfiram may increase phenytoin levels; baseline and periodic monitoring of phenytoin levels is recommended. Disulfiram also may prolong prothrombin time (PT) in patients concurrently prescribed oral anticoagulants. The drug should be used cautiously in patients with diabetes, hypothyroidism, epilepsy, nephritis, and hepatic dysfunction.

Naltrexone: The oral opioid μ-receptor antagonist naltrexone (ReVia™) is indicated for use in the treatment of alcohol dependence. Because alcohol is thought to indirectly increase activation of endogenous opioid receptors, blocking these receptors reduces the behavioral reinforcement and subsequently, the craving for alcohol. As compared with placebo-treated patients, those treated with naltrexone had lower relapse rates, fewer days of drinking, and less craving.[153] The dose of naltrexone as an adjunct to psychotherapy for alcohol dependence is 50 mg QD for up to 12 weeks. The drug is hepatotoxic and is contraindicated in patients with acute hepatitis or hepatic failure. Nausea, headache, and dizziness are common side effects. Patients treated with naltrexone cannot, of course, be treated with narcotic analgesics such as codeine or morphine.

COCAINE ABUSE AND DEPENDENCE

Except for amphetamines, cocaine is the most powerful positive reinforcer in humans.[154] Cocaine dependence usually develops quickly because of the rapid onset and short duration of intense, pleasurable effect; persons thus need to use the drug frequently to maintain the desired central nervous system (CNS) effects.[13] The financial implications of cocaine abuse or dependence are substantial because of the rapid stimulation provided by the drug and the need to obtain large sums of money in a brief period of time. The spread of sexually transmitted diseases, including AIDS, also becomes an issue when sexual promiscuity is exchanged for cocaine or for money to buy it.

Epidemiology

Exact figures for cocaine abuse and dependence are not known, but a 1991 survey estimates that 12% of the US population have used cocaine one or more times in their life. Cocaine misuse affects persons of every race, gender, and socioeconomic strata;[13] these disorders are equally common in males and females and are most prevalent in persons 30 years of age or younger. These disorders often are associated with abuse or dependence of other substances (eg, alcohol, benzodiazepines, marijuana), and also are frequently comorbid with PTSD and personality disorders.

Pathophysiology

- CNS effects are extensive

- ↑ Dopamine release and ↓ dopamine reuptake in brain areas involved in reward pathways (ie, pleasure center)

- Inhibits norepinephrine and serotonin reuptake as well as GABA and ACH.[155,156]

Presentation

Acute cocaine intoxication involves intense euphoria, increased energy, restlessness, talkativeness (rambling speech), anxiety, alertness, tactile hallucinations, and impaired judgment. Physical signs and symptoms include tachycardia or bradycardia, pupillary dilatation, elevated or low BP, perspiration or chills, and weakness. These may progress to respiratory depression, chest pain, arrhythmias, MI, stroke, confusion, seizures, or coma.[13] Persons dependent on cocaine often have transient mood symptoms during periods of withdrawal that meet criteria for major depression (see Table 14); many cocaine abusers seek medical help because of sexual dysfunction.[155]

Physical findings are linked to the route of cocaine administration. Sinusitis, nasal irritation or bleeding, or perforated nasal septum are found in those who "snort" cocaine. Respiratory problems such as coughing or bronchitis are common to those who smoke the substance. Puncture marks and forearm "tracks" are common to those who inject cocaine.[13] Weight loss is common because cocaine is an appetite suppressant.[155]

Diagnosis/Screening Tools

There are no specific diagnostic criteria for either cocaine abuse or dependence other than the general criteria (Tables 28 and 29). A urine test for a cocaine metabolite (benzoylecgonine) may identify recent cocaine use. This metabolite can be identified 1 to 3 days after a single dose and 7 to 12 days in persons using repeated, high doses.[13] The MINI (Part K; see APPENDIX) may be useful in the primary care setting.

Cocaine abuse and dependence cause far-ranging complications in nearly every body system.[155,157] Mildly elevated LFTs, hepatitis, tuberculosis, and sexually transmitted diseases (including AIDS) may be found in cocaine abusers. Mild pneumonitis or pneumothorax is sometimes found.

Referral

- Refer patients to self-help groups (eg, Cocaine Anonymous) or individual or group rehabilitation programs with experience in stimulant drug dependence.

Treatment

Pharmacologic treatment is highly specialized and remains second line to psychotherapeutic approaches or self-help groups (eg, Cocaine Anonymous). Antipsychotic drugs that act by blocking dopamine receptors (eg, haloperidol) may act as cocaine antagonists, and desipramine, carbamazepine, and dopamine agonists (eg, bromocriptine) have reduced craving, but data are limited and general recommendations for use of these drugs in primary care settings cannot be made.[147,154,155]

NICOTINE ABUSE AND DEPENDENCE

Nicotine dependence is estimated to occur in up to one half of the nearly 50 million US cigarette smokers; abstinence rates among those who attempt to quit smoking are very low — only 2% to 3% at 1 year.[158-160] Tobacco-related diseases claim the lives of half of all smokers; cigarette smoking is thought to be the most important preventable cause of death and disease in the US.[161] Also of paramount importance are illnesses related to second-hand or environmental smoke.

A number of prescription and nonprescription nicotine-replacement products are available to aid patients in smoking cessation (eg, nicotine nasal spray, nicotine chewing gum, nicotine transdermal patches). Readers are referred to comprehensive reviews for more information.[160] The following section focuses on the use of the antidepressant bupropion, which recently was approved in a sustained-release formulation (Zyban®) as the first non-nicotine aid for smoking cessation. Refer to page 93 for complete information on the side effects, contraindications, and drug interactions with bupropion.

Referral

- Numerous counseling and support services are available for persons wishing to stop smoking.[162]

Treatment

Sustained-release bupropion has been compared with placebo and transdermal nicotine (alone and in combination) and, although published data are limited, the manufacturer reports statistically significantly higher rates of smoking cessation with bupropion after 7 to 10 weeks of treatment. The exact mechanism of sustained-release bupropion for smoking cessation is not clear; as compared with TCAs, the drug is a weak norepinephrine and serotonin reuptake inhibitor. It also is a mild dopamine-receptor agonist; dopamine may play a role in "reward" or reinforcement behavior and norepinephrine may cause withdrawal symptoms[163] (also see Table 51). For smoking cessation, a dose of 150 mg is prescribed once daily for 3 days and then increased to 150 mg twice daily, if tolerated, for up to 12 weeks with or without supplemental nicotine replacement. Smoking cessation counseling should be continued. Patients should be advised to stop smoking during the second week of treatment, when steady-state bupropion levels have been attained. Long-term relapse rates are high with all smoking cessation aids including bupropion.[163]

OPIATE ABUSE AND DEPENDENCE

The opiate class includes natural (eg, morphine), semisynthetic (eg, heroin), and synthetic (eg, codeine, hydromorphone, meperidine, fentanyl, oxycodone) products. Opiates can be obtained through illegal methods or legally, as in cough suppressants, analgesics, and antidiarrheal agents.

Epidemiology

Exact incidence figures are not known, but it appears that opiate abuse is again on the rise. Approximately 6% of a community population reported ever using analgesics for nonmedical uses, although these data do not necessarily indicate a diagnosis of opiate abuse or dependence, only usage patterns.[13] There is little evidence supporting one hypothesis that treatment of medical or surgical patients with narcotic analgesics is associated with subsequent opiate abuse. Opiate misuse disorders usually appear in persons in their late teens to early 20s and are about three times more common in males. Dependence is usually chronic and relapse usually follows brief periods of abstinence. Opiate misuse disorders are associated with divorce, unemployment, or irregular employment.[13] Opiate-dependent patients are at risk for major depression, and these disorders are commonly comorbid with PTSD and personality disorders. Other important implications of opiate abuse or dependence include transmission of human immunodeficiency virus (HIV), tuberculosis, tetanus (rare), hepatitis, or endocarditis. The high mortality rates in opiate users are due to accidents, overdose, and injuries related to either use or procurement of the substance.

Pathophysiology

- May ↑ dopamine concentrations in areas of the brain involved with "reward" or reinforcement.[146]

Presentation

Individuals who are acutely intoxicated with an opiate have constricted pupils, drowsiness, slurred speech, impaired memory, and inattentiveness. Severe intoxication may produce coma, respiratory depression, pinpoint pupils, or death. Other physical signs of acute or chronic opiate dependence are reduced oral and nasal secretions, constipation, or impaired vision (due to constricted pupils). In intravenous (IV) opiate users, tracks (sclerosed veins) will be present on the extremities.

Most opiate-dependent individuals have a high degree of tolerance and experience withdrawal symptoms (eg, anxiety, restlessness, achy feeling, opiate craving, irritability) when the substance is acutely withdrawn.[13] Elevated LFTs are common.

Diagnosis/Screening Tools

There are no specific diagnostic criteria other than those in Tables 28 and 29; urine tests for opiates can detect current opiate use. Hepatitis screening tests often are positive.

Referral

- Refer all patients with opiate dependence to specialized facilities for psychotherapy, methadone maintenance, or other detoxification or withdrawal programs (such clinics are licensed by the FDA and the Drug Enforcement Agency [DEA])
- Self-help groups (eg, Narcotics Anonymous) are also effective and may be of interest to the patient.

Treatment

There are many treatment programs for opiate-dependent patients, but few patients are ultimately cured. Most patients focus on self-improvement while dealing with chronic opiate dependence by receiving chronic maintenance therapy. Maintenance programs and the physicians who direct them must be licensed to prescribe and dispense methadone or LAAM (see below) by the FDA and the DEA. Acute detoxification and maintenance regimens must be individualized; treatment protocols have not been developed and are not recommended for these disorders.

Methadone: For more than 30 years, short-term substitution therapy with oral methadone (Dolophine®) has been the main pharmacologic approach for opiate dependence.[144] Acutely, methadone is used to suppress withdrawal signs and symptoms and then is gradually tapered entirely or to a level considered maintenance therapy (ie, 20 or 40 mg QD) while patients undergo psychotherapy and other efforts to improve their overall health. In the inpatient setting, methadone tapering can be performed over a relatively short time (1 or 2 weeks), whereas in the outpatient setting, it is accomplished over several months.

LAAM: A newer product, LAAM (ORLAAM®, L-α-acetyl-methadol, levomethadyl acetate), is a long-acting methadone analog approved only for maintenance treatment of opiate dependence. It is given every other day or three times weekly.[144]

Miscellaneous: Buprenorphine, a partial opioid agonist, can be given sublingually for prevention of withdrawal symptoms.[164] The α-adrenergic agonists clonidine, lofexidine, guanabenz, and guanfacine also are effective in this regard for some patients and are not addicting. Naltrexone, an opioid-receptor antagonist (see page 50), has been useful in preventing relapse in some opiate-dependent persons (reviewed in reference 144).[164]

Eating Disorders

Both anorexia nervosa (AN) and bulimia nervosa (BN) are characterized by severely disordered eating behavior caused by altered perception of body shape and weight.[13] Most patients display both anorectic and bulimic behaviors and are concerned with body weight and becoming fat. However, only those with AN successfully lower body weight on a long-term basis, often to life-threatening levels.[165] Unfortunately, drug therapy has a very limited role in AN. At least 90% of eating disorder cases occur in women. Prevalence rates are higher in certain groups such as models, actresses, athletes, and dancers.[166]

ANOREXIA NERVOSA

AN is a chronic, serious condition characterized by severe weight loss and a refusal or failure to maintain a minimally normal body weight. Weight loss is accomplished through restricted food intake (individuals first exclude high-calorie foods but typically end up with a very limited and restrictive diet), by purging, or by increased or excessive exercise.[13] Although implied, loss of appetite (anorexia) is rare in AN; however, the initial weight loss may be preceded by loss of appetite caused by depression, illness,[167] or dieting.

Epidemiology

AN is relatively rare (0.5% to 1% prevalence in late-adolescent or early-adult females; more common in industrialized societies),[166] and it has increased in the past 3 or 4 decades. Few data are available in males. AN often starts with dieting and a stressful life event; the mean age at onset is 17 years and it is rare in women older than 40 years of age. There is an increased risk for AN in first-degree female relatives of patients with the disorder. The course is variable; it may be limited to only one episode, or it may be fluctuating or chronic and deteriorating. Mortality among individuals admitted to university hospitals is higher than 10%; death results from starvation, suicide, or electrolyte imbalance leading to cardiac arrhythmia. AN is often comorbid with major depression (50% to 75% of cases[168]), OCD (if obsessions and compulsions are unrelated to food), or substance abuse.

Pathophysiology

- Serotonin dysregulation implicated;[169] serotonin is integral in feeding and satiety behaviors, behavioral and mood disorders, and regulation of other neurotransmitters (eg, CRF, TRH, CCK)

- In contrast to BN, AN may be a hyperserotonergic state, which could ↑ satiety and ↓ food intake.[165]

Presentation

Individuals with AN rarely complain of weight loss as a symptom (indeed, they typically deny the problem) but are concerned with physical manifestations of semistarvation (eg, bloated feeling, constipation, abdominal pain, being cold and intolerant to cold temperatures, and either lethargy or excessive energy). The patient may appear depressed, withdrawn, or irritable. Parents or friends offer a more reliable history; the patient may admit to being preoccupied or obsessed with thoughts of food. Persons may complain of feeling fat overall or may be concerned that certain body parts (eg, thighs, abdomen) are fat even though the patient realizes that they are thin. Weight loss is a significant achievement, whereas weight gain represents a loss of self-control.

On physical exam, the patient appears emaciated because of the loss of subcutaneous fat and up to 60% of total body weight. Prepubertal females may show arrested physical and sexual maturation. Hypotension is common (systolic blood pressure <70 mm Hg). The skin may be dry or yellow (hyper-carotenemia); petechiae on the extremities may indicate a bleeding diathesis or increased capillary permeability. Lanugo (fine silky hair covering the trunk and extremities) may be present. Peripheral edema may develop during a phase of weight gain or when diuretic or laxative abuse is stopped. Teeth may be mottled due to erosion of enamel from induced vomiting. Abnormal laboratory findings (Table 31) are related to starvation.[13]

Table 31. Abnormal laboratory findings in AN[13]

Test	Findings
Hematology	Leukopenia with relative lymphocytosis, mild normochromic normocytic anemia, thrombocytopenia (rare)
Chemistry	↑ BUN, ↑ cholesterol, ↑ LFTs, ↓ Mg^{++}, ↓ PO_4, ↓ Zn, ↓ K^+, metabolic alkalosis (if ↑ vomiting) or acidosis (if laxative abuse), ↑ serum amylase, normal to ↓ T_4, ↓ T_3, ↓ serum estrogen (females)/testosterone (males), ↑ cortisol, hypoglycemia, glucose intolerance
ECG	Sinus bradycardia, murmurs, arrhythmias (rare)
EEG	Diffuse changes reflect metabolic encephalopathy
CT	↑ Ventricular-brain ratio (pseudoatrophy)

Abbreviations defined in GLOSSARY.

Diagnosis/Screening Tools

Diagnostic criteria for AN are shown in Table 32.[13] The MINI (Part M; see APPENDIX) contains useful information on screening for AN.

Normal weight should be assessed using published charts (eg, Metropolitan Life Insurance tables, Iowa Growth Chart). Patients with AN should be classified as either bulimic subtype (binge-eating/purging) or restricting subtype (nonbulimic). The former often resembles BN.

Table 32. Diagnostic criteria for AN (adapted from reference 13, with permission).
© Copyright 1994, American Psychiatric Association.

- Refusal to maintain body weight at or above minimal normal cutoff for age and height (eg, weight loss or failure to make expected weight gains during a growth phase → body weight <85% of expected)
- Intense fear of gaining weight or becoming fat even though underweight
- Disturbed perception of body shape or weight, denial of seriousness of low body weight
- Amenorrhea: absence of ≥3 menstrual cycles in a postmenarchal female

Abbreviations defined in GLOSSARY.

Panhypopituitarism or medical causes of weight loss (eg, cancer, GI disease, AIDS) should be ruled out, although individuals who are suffering from weight loss because of medical reasons usually do not have the distorted sense of body shape or size that those with AN have. AN should be differentiated from eating disorders or weight loss that may occur in schizophrenia, major depression, or social anxiety disorder (eg, fear of eating in public). Depressive features may be secondary to physiologic complications of starvation and therefore should be assessed further after partial or complete restoration of weight.[13]

Referral

- Refer patients with suspected eating disorders for nutritional rehabilitation and individual and family psychotherapy
- Hospitalize severely underweight patients (<80% of expected body weight) for stabilization of electrolyte and other physiologic sequelae.

Treatment

Treatment goals are initially focused on restoration of a normal (or minimally normal) body weight and correction of physiologic and biologic sequelae of malnutrition/starvation. Longer-term goals are to initiate psychotherapy or behavioral therapy to correct poor eating habits and prevent relapse. Highly motivated patients can be treated as outpatients with close monitoring by those skilled in eating disorders.

Drugs have a very limited role in the routine management of AN because of lack of evidence for efficacy and because the documented neurotransmitter dysregulations are almost always normalized with proper nutritional rehabilitation. Thus, a psychopharmacologic treatment algorithm is not provided for AN. There are few controlled data on the use of psychopharmacologic agents in the treatment of AN, and no class or agent has shown consistent benefit. Use of antipsychotic drugs (eg, chlorpromazine) to manage obsessional behavior is uncommon today. Severely malnourished patients may be more prone to psychotropic drug-induced side effects.[168] Anxiolytics may be useful in managing meal-related anxiety although controlled data are lacking. Historically, antidepressants were used because of the side effect of weight gain;[170] they can be effective in treating comorbid depression, however. Limited anecdotal data with low-dose fluoxetine have shown some benefit in restoring and maintaining weight. However, severely malnourished or dehydrated AN patients may be at greater risk for antidepressant side effects such as hypotension or arrhythmias. Depressed AN patients also may respond less well to antidepressant therapy than depressed patients without AN.[168]

BULIMIA NERVOSA

BN is characterized by repeated episodes of binge eating followed by inappropriate compensatory behaviors (eg, self-induced purging, fasting, or excessive exercise; rarely ipecac or thyroid hormone) to prevent weight gain. Unlike in AN, the patient with BN can maintain a minimally normal weight.

A *binge* is eating in a discrete period of time (usually <2 h) an amount of food larger than what most individuals would eat under similar circumstances.[13] Snacking throughout the day is not binge eating. Foods consumed during binges are usually sweet, high-calorie items. Binge eating is usually done in secrecy and is accompanied by feelings of shame.

Epidemiology

BN is more common than AN and the number of cases has risen during the past few decades. BN affects 1% to 3% of young (usually Caucasian) women and approximately 0.1% to 0.3% of males.[13,166] The onset is in late adolescence or early adulthood and a genetic component is likely. Binge eating may follow an episode of dieting as a means to reduce hunger. The course may be chronic or intermittent.[171] Within 5 to 10 years after presentation, 20% of women still meet diagnostic criteria for BN; 50% will experience full recovery.[171] BN frequently is comorbid with depression, anxiety disorders, substance abuse, or personality disorders.[168]

Pathophysiology

- Cause not fully known, but brain serotonin synthesis may be ↓ (ie, a hyposerotonergic state), which would lead to ↓ satiety and ↑ food intake[165]

- Dietary restriction may lead to ↓ plasma tryptophan and further ↓ serotonin. Food intake also is controlled by other neurotransmitters (eg, norepinephrine) and neuropeptides (NPY, CCK, galanin)

- Possible role of social factors (eg, an ideal woman is thin) not yet clarified.

Presentation

As in AN, patients with BN are dissatisfied with their body shape and fear becoming overweight. Individuals with this disorder are ashamed of their binging behavior and try to conceal it. Binge eating continues until the individual is painfully full; between binges, the individual consumes low-calorie foods. Two subtypes of BN are described: the purging subtype, in which self-induced vomiting or medication abuse (laxatives, enemas, diuretics) is common, and the nonpurging subtype, in which fasting or exercise is the preferred method of weight control.

On physical examination, the patient is usually within a normal weight range (but may be slightly below or above it) but shows physiologic signs of starvation. If purging is present, there will be a loss of dental enamel and chipped or ragged front teeth; these patients usually are cavity prone. Parotid salivary glands are enlarged. Menstrual irregularities can occur. Resting bradycardia, hypotension, and decreased metabolic rate may occur. Some patients may be dependent on laxatives. Rare but possible complications more common in the BN purging subtype are esophageal tears, gastric rupture due to acute gastric dilatation, or arrhythmias.

Laboratory abnormalities include hypokalemia, hyponatremia, hypochloremia, mild hyperamylasemia, metabolic alkalosis (in frequent purgers), or acidosis (in laxative abusers). If the patient abuses ipecac, cardiomyopathy or peripheral muscle weakness may be present.

Diagnosis/Screening Tools

The patient and family members should be interviewed to obtain historical information that may contribute to the diagnosis of BN (Table 33). The MINI (Part N; see APPENDIX) contains useful screening information. Overeating may be part of other psychiatric disorders (eg, major depression) except that compensatory behavior is not present.

Table 33. Diagnostic criteria for BN (adapted from reference 13, with permission). © Copyright 1994, American Psychiatric Association.

- Recurrent episodes of binge eating and a sense of lack of control during the episode
- Recurrent, inappropriate compensatory behavior to prevent weight gain
  - self-induced vomiting
  - abuse of laxatives, diuretics, enemas
  - fasting
  - excessive exercise
- Binge eating and compensatory behaviors occur about twice weekly for 3 months but do not occur exclusively during an episode of AN
- Self-evaluation is unduly influenced by body shape and weight

---

Abbreviations defined in GLOSSARY.

Referral

- For maximum benefit, refer the patient and family members for nutritional counseling, behavioral therapy, psychotherapy, and drug therapy.

Treatment

As in AN, treatment goals in BN are focused on restoration of a normal (or minimally normal) body weight and correction of physiologic and biologic sequelae of malnutrition/starvation. For the longer term, CBT can be used to correct poor eating habits and prevent relapse. Used in conjunction with CBT, antidepressants reduce the number of binge episodes and bulimic symptoms in BN patients regardless of whether they are depressed.[165,168,172] The TCAs,[173] SSRIs,[174] MAOIs, and trazodone have been shown to be effective. Doses of TCAs and MAOIs are the same as for depression; higher SSRI doses may be more effective (eg, fluoxetine 60 mg QD often is recommended for treatment of BN). MAOIs must be used carefully because of the need for a tyramine-free diet. Several different antidepressants may need to be tried before benefit is achieved; bupropion is contraindicated in eating disorders because of risk of seizures. If a patient is not responding to one antidepressant after 2 or 3 weeks, plasma-level monitoring may provide confirmation that the dose is not being taken or is being affected by purging. Little is known about the optimal duration of treatment because long-term data are not available.

Dementia of the Alzheimer's Type

Dementia of the Alzheimer's type, or Alzheimer's disease (AD), is the most common primary, progressive, degenerative dementia in the elderly and the fourth leading cause of death in the US.[175,176] At an annual cost of more than $90 billion in the US alone, AD has important public health implications, especially in concert with the unparalleled growth of the aged population.[175,177]

Epidemiology

AD afflicts up to 4 million US adults,[175] a figure that may double by the year 2000. The prevalence clearly increases with age; up to 50% of US adults older than 85 years may have the disorder.[178,179] Overall estimates of the incidence of AD (1%/y) are hindered by a lack of reliable data.[175] AD greatly reduces life expectancy; median survival is 5 to 8 years after diagnosis,[175] but the illness can persist for up to 20 years until death.[180] Life expectancy is lower in men than in women and in those with significantly impaired cognition at the time of diagnosis. Risk factors for AD are shown in Table 34.[175]

Table 34. Possible risk factors for AD[175,181,182]

Risk factor	Comments
Aluminum	Unresolved; ↑ aluminosilicate levels found in NFT and plaques of patients with AD but aluminum inhalation or ingestion (eg, aluminum-containing antacids) does not cause AD
Apolipoprotein E4	Presence of the E4 allele is a strong risk factor for late-onset AD but not diagnostic
Cigarette smoking	Positive and negative (protective) associations reported
Diet	Delayed onset of dementia in vegetarians versus heavy meat eaters reported but needs replication
Education level	AD occurs more often in undereducated persons
Estrogen deficiency	↑ Risk in postmenopausal women not using estrogen supplements
Family history	Positive family history ↑ risk
Female gender	Unresolved whether women are at ↑ risk
Head injury	Head trauma with loss of consciousness or retrograde amnesia may ↑ risk of AD in men in later life
Maternal age	Late maternal age may ↑ risk of AD in offspring
Thyroid disease	Unconfirmed association
Trisomy 21 (Down syndrome)	Similar neuropathologic and cognitive features of AD; relatives may be at ↑ risk for AD

Abbreviations defined in GLOSSARY.

Pathophysiology

- Unknown cause, but genetic component is certain in familial form and likely in other forms[183]
- Primary degenerative CNS changes include prominent cerebral atrophy in cortical association areas, neuronal losses, neurofibrillary tangles (NFT), and neuritic or senile ß-amyloid plaques (latter two are hallmark neurohistologic lesions)
- Neurotransmitter deficits resulting from these degenerative changes include ACH, and dopamine, norepinephrine, serotonin, somatostatin, CRF, and GABA
- ↓ ACH caused by degeneration of cholinergic neurons in the basal forebrain resulting in ↓ activity of enzymes involved in ACH synthesis (choline acetyltransferase [ChAT]) and degradation (acetylcholinesterase).[184]

Presentation

Insidious memory loss in someone older than 65 years of age is the hallmark feature of AD although patients have been identified with earlier-onset memory loss (eg, 40 to 65 years); short-term memory loss occurs in early AD and is eventually followed by long-term memory loss.[185] Patients become progressively unable to perform activities of daily living and personal hygiene functions. At least 40% of patients with AD develop disruptive, agitated behavior (eg, physical or verbal abuse, aggression, agitation, screaming, wandering, uncooperativeness) that may adversely affect cognitive function (ie, by interfering with motivation or attentiveness)[176] as well as the overall management of AD. Hallucinations and delusions usually appear during the early or middle stages of the disorder. In contrast to the more complex, grandiose delusions of schizophrenia, delusions of AD are usually simple, paranoid beliefs related to memory loss. Typical delusions include perceived theft of money or personal items, a belief that a long-deceased acquaintance is still alive, or that one's spouse is an impostor (Capgras' syndrome). These differences between delusions of schizophrenia and those of AD may explain why antipsychotic drugs are less effective in the latter disorder.

Depression often coexists with AD and can aggravate simple memory loss. In advanced AD, patients have profound dementia and aphasia and usually are bedridden, incontinent, and unable to remain alone or in a home setting without constant care.

Diagnosis/Screening Tools

The National Institute of Neurological and Communicative Disorders and Stroke and the Alzheimer's Disease and Related Disorders Association (NINCDS-ADRDA) task force has established commonly used diagnostic criteria for possible, probable, or definite AD.[186] Although a definitive diagnosis of AD currently can only be made on autopsy or brain biopsy, measurement of abnormal concentrations of certain proteins in cerebrospinal fluid (CSF) shows promise as a diagnostic test.[187] Diagnostic criteria according to the DSM-IV are provided in Table 35.

Table 35. Diagnostic criteria for AD (adapted from reference 13, with permission). © Copyright 1994, American Psychiatric Association.

- Multiple cognitive defects that cause significant impairment in social or occupational function:
  - memory impairment
  - cognitive disturbances (eg, language disorders [aphasia], impaired motor abilities [apraxia], inability to recognize objects [agnosia], disturbed executive functioning [eg, planning, concentration, organizing])
- Characterized by gradual and continuing cognitive decline
- Psychiatric, neurologic, or systemic conditions that might adversely affect memory or cause dementia have been ruled out

Abbreviations defined in GLOSSARY.

AD is only one possible diagnosis in an older individual with reduced cognitive function. Other dementing illnesses such as Pick's disease or supranuclear palsy must be ruled out. Other causes of impaired memory loss such as that due to normal aging processes, encephalopathies (eg, from anoxia, head trauma), vascular or multi-infarct dementia, or an acute confusional state related to a metabolic, toxic (drugs, alcohol), or infectious disorder must be ruled out.[182]

To establish progressive deterioration in memory and cognitive skills, a careful evaluation must be performed, including a detailed family history with an informant other than the patient, medication history, past medical history, and a complete physical, neuropsychologic, and laboratory workup (Table 36). Referral for structural neuroimaging studies (eg, magnetic resonance imaging [MRI], computed tomography [CT]) is useful.[182,186,188]

In the office setting, the Mini Mental State Examination (MMSE),[189] Blessed Dementia Scale,[190] or Short Portable Mental Status Questionnaire[191] may be used to screen a patient in whom dementia is suspected. On the MMSE, a score of 26 or less is abnormal in a high school graduate, and a score of 27 to 30 with evidence of cognitive decline should prompt more detailed neuropsychologic testing.[192] If clinical suspicion is raised, more detailed neuropsychologic testing should be conducted as outlined by the NINCDS-ADRDA.[186] Patients with AD show a reduction of 3 to 4 points/y on the Blessed Memory Concentration Test or a reduction of 2 to 3 points/y on the MMSE with each year of illness.

Table 36. Diagnostic approach to the patient with suspected AD[182,186]

Evaluation	Goal	Approach
Medical	Establish history of progressive memory loss and inability to perform tasks	Interview patient, family, close acquaintances. Obtain detailed family, medication (prescription, OTC), and past medical history (eg, stroke, seizure, head trauma, psychiatric)
Clinical	Document diagnostic inclusion and exclusion criteria	Perform physical examination, mental status testing (eg, MMSE), neurologic testing
Laboratory	Enhance diagnostic accuracy	Obtain routine blood, electrolyte, renal, liver, metabolic studies; also, vitamin B_{12}, folic acid, TFTs, ESR, syphilis or HIV (if risk factors present)
Neuropsychologic[a]	Provide additional information on diagnosis of dementia	Recognition Span Test, Boston Naming Test, Wechsler Adult Intelligence Scale, Continuous Performance Test, Gollin Incomplete Pictures Test, Wisconsin Card Sorting Test, Philadelphia Geriatrics Center forms
Neuroimaging	Identify potentially treatable causes of dementia (eg, tumor, abscess, subdural hematoma)	CT or MRI
	Identify ↓ regional glucose metabolism and blood flow in parietal and temporal lobes	PET or SPECT (mainly research tools)

Abbreviations defined in GLOSSARY.
[a]See reference 186 for more detailed information.

Referral

- Refer patient to psychiatrist if AD complicated by psychosis or severe depression
- Refer family members or caregivers to local support services (see RESOURCES) to alleviate stresses associated with care of the patient with AD.

Treatment

Because AD is a chronic, progressive disorder, by necessity, treatment approaches must be customized and continually adjusted according to the patient's current situation.[180,193] A multidisciplinary approach to address medical, social, psychological, and environmental issues involves both nonpharmacologic and pharmacologic avenues.[178]

Nonpharmacologic approaches include behavioral counseling for patients and caregivers and home safety evaluation (eg, provide living arrangements on a single level of the home to eliminate need to use stairs, enhance lighting in dark hallways, lower hot water temperature, eliminate throw rugs, torn carpeting, slippery surfaces). Family members and caregivers themselves often become "second patients"; about 80% of spousal caregivers experience clinically significant anxiety or depressive symptoms and more frequent medical illness associated with chronic stress during the course of AD.[180]

Currently available pharmacotherapy (Figure 9) cannot delay or prevent the onset of AD, but rather is directed at restoring primary underlying neurotransmitter deficits (ie, low central ACH levels). However, one of the most active ongoing research programs is directed toward development of agents that will prevent or reduce amyloid formation in patients with AD.[177] Currently, only tacrine (see page 152) and donepezil (see page 155) are approved in the US for the treatment of the dementia of AD. Ergoloid mesylates (see page 151) have been used in elderly demented patients but with little clinical success. Selegiline (see page 156) also may improve cognition and inappropriate behavior. Other new compounds are actively being studied.[184,194]

Pharmacotherapy also can be directed at managing secondary behavioral disturbances such as aggression or agitation, depression, or psychosis (Figure 9).[185]

Antipsychotics: Much of the data supporting antipsychotic use in elderly patients with AD has been extrapolated from studies in younger, demented patients. More randomized clinical trials are needed in elderly patients with NINCDS-ADRDA-defined AD. Antipsychotics have demonstrated limited efficacy over placebo for the cardinal features of AD.[185,195] According to a meta-analysis, no antipsychotic drug offers substantial clinical advantage over another; therefore, drug selection should be made based on potential side effects (eg, highly anticholinergic agents may worsen cognition). Antipsychotics are most effective for managing classic psychotic symptoms (eg, grandiose, complex delusions) and less effective in patients who are not agitated, hyperactive, or not experiencing hallucinations or delusions (Table 37).[176]

Figure 9. Pharmacologic treatment approach to the patient with AD.[178] Abbreviations defined in GLOSSARY.

EVALUATE and examine patient:
Family/medical/drug history
Laboratory/neurologic testing

INTERVIEW reliable family member/acquaintance

INITIATE pharmacologic therapy:
- Restore neurotransmitter deficits: tacrine, donepezil
- Improve cognition: selegiline, ergoloid mesylates

ASSESS bothersome secondary behavioral disturbances:
Depression
Antidepressants (eg, SSRIs, trazodone, nortriptyline, venlafaxine, nefazodone)
Psychosis
Antipsychotics: typical (eg, haloperidol) or atypical (eg, clozapine, olanzapine, risperidone, quetiapine)
Agitation/Violent Behavior
Antipsychotics (as above)
Anticonvulsants (eg, carbamazepine, valproic acid)
Anxiolytics (eg, buspirone, benzodiazepines)
Antidepressants

MONITOR:
Therapeutic benefit, tolerability → ADJUST dose if needed

CONSIDER:
- Benefit and need for continued drug therapy; consider discontinuing antipsychotic after 3 months to avoid long-term exposure (EPS)
- Need to change therapeutic approach for emergence of new symptoms
- Psychiatric referral for difficult or nonresponding cases

Table 37. Secondary behavioral symptoms of AD and expected response to psychopharmacologic intervention[193]

• More likely to respond	Nonspecific hyperactivity, physical or verbal agitation, classic psychoses or delusions, depressive symptoms, hallucinations
• Less likely to respond	Wandering, public disrobing, hoarding or hiding objects and possessions, repetitive questioning, social inappropriateness

Abbreviations defined in GLOSSARY.

Because functional improvements often are limited by excess sedation and extrapyramidal side effects (EPS), clinicians should consider the impact of antipsychotic therapy on the quality of life of the AD patient and his or her caregivers. Clearly the newer atypical antipsychotics such as risperidone, olanzapine, and quetiapine will have a major role here. Generally, these are initiated at low doses (eg, 0.5 to 1 mg risperidone, 2.5 mg olanzapine) to avoid side effects. If the patient and caregiver can tolerate certain disruptive behavior, antipsychotic drug therapy could be withheld, at least temporarily. On the other hand, psychotic symptoms may be associated with faster cognitive deterioration.[185]

Antidepressants: Antidepressants have not been well studied in depressed patients with AD, and the response to placebo is very high.[196] Thus, early *response* to an antidepressant may forecast an early *relapse.* Antidepressants may improve mood or disturbed sleep-wake cycles, but they have no effect on cognitive functioning unless the patient is suffering from depressive pseudodementia. A low dose of an antidepressant such as an SSRI or one of the newer atypical antidepressants should be selected. TCAs should be avoided because of their adverse cardiac effects and anticholinergic properties, but if necessary, a secondary amine TCA (eg, nortriptyline, desipramine) can be used and the dose gradually increased. If improvement is not noted after adequate doses are given for an appropriate period of time, another agent should be chosen. Plasma levels considered therapeutic in nondemented depressed individuals may not apply to demented depressed patients.[196]

Anticonvulsants: Results of numerous open[197,198] and small, nonrandomized, placebo-controlled studies[199] have shown that carbamazepine, in doses of 100 to 300 mg/d (plasma levels 4 to 12 µg/mL), is well tolerated and effectively alleviates agitated, disruptive, or aggressive behavior in patients with AD who have not responded to antipsychotic drugs. Similarly, valproic acid also has been shown to be effective in this population (plasma levels of 50 to 60 ng/mL),[200] although it has not been as thoroughly examined in controlled trials.[201] Neither of these agents should be considered first-line treatment for the management of agitation in patients with AD, but could be considered for nonresponsive, nonpsychotic, mildly agitated patients.[178]

Schizophrenia

Schizophrenia is the most common of the psychotic disorders.[202] The societal impact includes issues of unemployment, homelessness, and direct and indirect costs probably exceeding $75 billion annually.[203]

Epidemiology

The lifetime prevalence of schizophrenia is approximately 1%; prevalence rates worldwide are similar. Schizophrenia generally begins in late adolescence or early adulthood; the median age at onset in men (early 20s) is slightly earlier than in women (late 20s). Men and women are affected equally. The course is variable; some patients experience exacerbations and remissions (although full remission is rare), whereas others remain chronically ill. Extensive family and twin genetic studies show schizophrenia to be more common in family members of affected individuals, although it can arise spontaneously. Suicide occurs in 10% to 13% of schizophrenic patients and is attempted by 18% to 55%.[203] Schizophrenia is commonly comorbid with substance abuse disorders, especially alcohol. After successful treatment of a first episode, the risk of relapse is approximately 40% to 60% in patients not on maintenance treatment.[203]

Pathophysiology

- Genetics have a role but environmental (obstetrical) factors (eg, Rh incompatibility, in utero exposure to influenza virus or malnutrition) are also likely to be important[202]

- Focal brain lesions that develop before birth may cause alterations in many neurotransmitter systems

- Early research focused on the "dopaminergic hypothesis," but many neurotransmitters are now known to be involved; complex interactions between them have not yet been elucidated (eg, in schizophrenia, dopamine [D_2] receptors are ↑; dopamine is partially modulated by serotonin, which supports the clinical utility of atypical antipsychotics [see page 136] that preferentially block serotonin [$5\text{-}HT_2$] receptors)[204]

- Glutamate transmission may be abnormal (glutamate ↑ GABA whereas dopamine ↓ GABA).[202]

Presentation

Schizophrenia comprises a cluster of positive (ie, excessive or distorted normal functioning), negative (ie, loss of normal functioning), cognitive, and mood symptoms (Table 38) that have a devastating effect on a patient's social, personal/interpersonal, and occupational functioning.[205]

Negative symptoms (see Table 38) usually develop first; these tend to be more chronic and treatment resistant and are soon followed by positive symptoms. Negative symptoms may be confused with depression or EPS.[206] At presentation, an individual may have an inappropriate affect (eg, laughing without an appropriate stimulus), depression or anxiety, sleep disturbances, motor abnormalities (eg, pacing), or difficulty concentrating or focusing. Lack of insight may predict poor outcome partly because it adversely affects patient compliance with therapy.[13] Schizophrenia may be easily confused with acute mania, psychotic depression, delusional disorders, or substance abuse (eg, cocaine, phencyclidine, LSD).[207]

Table 38. Core symptom clusters in schizophrenia

Symptom cluster	Examples
Positive	Delusions, hallucinations, disorganized (incoherent) speech, catatonia
Negative	Flat affect, alogia (paucity of speech), avolition (lack of goal-directed behavior), anhedonia (lack of enjoyment)
Cognitive	Attention and memory deficits, difficulty with abstract thinking
Mood	Dysphoria, suicidal thoughts, hopelessness

Diagnosis/Screening Tools

Diagnostic criteria for schizophrenia are shown in Table 39. Five schizophrenia subtypes are described in more detail in DSM-IV.[13]

Table 39. Diagnostic criteria for schizophrenia (adapted from reference 13, with permission). © Copyright 1994, American Psychiatric Association.

- ≥2 characteristic active-phase symptoms[a], present most of the time during a 1-month period:
  - delusions
  - hallucinations
  - disorganized (incoherent or loosely associated) speech
  - grossly disorganized or catatonic behavior
  - negative symptoms (see Table 38)
- Social or occupational dysfunction
- Continuous signs persist for ≥6 months. During this time, active-phase symptoms have been present for ≥1 month
- Substance abuse or direct physiologic effects of a general medical condition have been ruled out

[a]Only one symptom required if bizarre delusions (see GLOSSARY) or hallucinations involving conversing voices are present.

Patients should undergo a complete psychiatric and medical workup, mental status examination, and a physical exam including neurologic workup. Basic laboratory studies, including drug screen,[203] should be conducted. The risk of injury to the patient and to others should be carefully evaluated. No laboratory tests are diagnostic for schizophrenia. However, some individuals may have psychosis-induced polydipsia (drinking 4 to 10 L/d of water) that may cause hyponatremia.[13] On physical exam, some individuals may appear physically awkward and may show left/right confusion and poor coordination. Minor physical anomalies have been noted in schizophrenic individuals (eg, highly arched palate, subtle ear malformations, narrow- or wide-set eyes). Motor abnormalities (ie, EPS) may be prominent and related to antipsychotic drug therapy.[13]

If indicated, brain MRI or CT may show characteristic anatomic findings such as enlargement of cerebral ventricles and decreased brain volume. These findings are not related to the duration of illness or previous treatment but may predict poorer outcome to antipsychotic drug therapy.[202,203]

Referral

- Hospitalize severely or acutely ill schizophrenic patients who pose a significant safety risk to themselves or others. Hospitalize patients experiencing their first psychotic episode for safety, evaluation, and workup of new-onset psychosis

- Refer patients and family members for psychosocial counseling to improve their understanding of the disease, ways to maintain or improve compliance with the treatment plan, and ways to promote coping and independent functioning

- Most primary care physicians refer partially or totally treatment-resistant patients for psychiatric reassessment.

Treatment

Drug therapy is the mainstay of treatment for schizophrenia (Figure 10), but patient- and family-focused education about the recurring nature of the disorder may reduce the frequency of episodes and provide understanding about the rationale for drug treatment and potential side effects (eg, EPS).[203,208,209] Primary care physicians can have tremendous impact during all phases of treatment by acting as a liaison with the patient's other healthcare providers or family members and by promoting compliance with drug therapy. Noncompliance may be caused by denial of the illness, dissatisfaction with care providers, poor social support, substance abuse, and side effects,[207] and likely will result in recurrence of psychotic symptoms. Primary care physicians probably will have most contact with less severely ill patients who might require initiation of antipsychotic therapy, dose adjustments, or plasma-level monitoring, or with those who are receiving maintenance treatment.

Figure 10. Pharmacologic treatment approach to the patient with schizophrenia.[203,206,209]
Abbreviations defined in GLOSSARY.

EVALUATE and examine patient:
Severity of episode
Patient safety and risk of harm to others

CONSIDER patient features:
Ability to tolerate side effects
Previous response
Patient preference
Expected degree of compliance

INITIATE pharmacologic therapy:
- Typical antipsychotic: high potency (eg, haloperidol) or low potency (eg, chlorpromazine)
- Atypical antipsychotic: risperidone, quetiapine, or olanzapine
- Benzodiazepine for short-term management of insomnia or acute agitation, if needed

ASSESS tolerability after several days and response after 3 weeks. Plasma-level monitoring may be helpful to assess compliance, side-effect issues

Side effects:
- *Present, tolerable:* use lowest effective dose, add anticholinergic (eg, trihexyphenidyl, benztropine) or antihistamine (eg, diphenhydramine), if needed
- *Intolerable:* choose alternate antipsychotic with different side-effect profile

Response:
- *Acceptable:* continue antipsychotic at lowest effective dose. Maintain 12 - 24 months
- *Partial:* ↑ dose, continue several more weeks, assess response
- *None:* choose alternate antipsychotic agent

CONSIDER:
- Postpsychotic depression: add SSRI or TCA (see Figure 6)
- Substance abuse issues: referral to substance abuse program
- Psychiatric referral for difficult or severely ill patients, those continuing to have intolerable side effects, nonresponse of positive psychotic symptoms after ≥6 weeks of an adequate antipsychotic dose

Acute Phase: Antipsychotics: The goals of acute treatment are to reduce symptoms, prevent harm to or by the patient, improve the level of functioning, and establish short- and long-term treatment plans. Typical neuroleptic drugs (eg, chlorpromazine, haloperidol) have traditionally been first-line treatment for schizophrenia (Figure 10); they are similarly effective and drug selection can be based on the desired pharmacologic profile (eg, a more sedating agent may be preferred for an anxious patient) (see Table 80). Atypical antipsychotics risperidone, quetiapine, or olanzapine also are acceptable (and in some cases preferred) for first-line oral treatment because the risks of EPS are low; clozapine is restricted for use only in treatment-resistant patients (see page 137). Other factors to consider when choosing therapy include previous response, patient preference, and expected degree of compliance (ie, if the patient may eventually be given a long-acting depot injection, the clinician may select the corresponding oral formulation of the drug).[203]

Antipsychotic therapy should be initiated with low doses (see Tables 80 and 84) and titrated upward as needed after about 3 weeks. Use of high initial doses (ie, *rapid neuroleptization*) is not appropriate because it is associated with significant side effects.[203] Plasma-level monitoring may be useful to assess compliance, but a relation between level and therapeutic response has not been conclusively demonstrated for most antipsychotics. If patient compliance is a problem, liquid formulations or depot injections should be considered. Side effects (EPS) can be managed by adding anticholinergic or antihistaminic drugs as discussed in DRUGS FOR EXTRAPYRAMIDAL SIDE EFFECTS (see page 145).

Most patients will respond if antipsychotic therapy is prescribed in appropriate doses for an adequate duration (ie, ≥6 weeks).[207] Patients who have responded to antipsychotic therapy likely will respond similarly during future psychotic episodes. However, in some patients, the response diminishes with successive episodes. Features that may predict a more favorable outcome include female gender, late onset, good premorbid functioning, acute (versus insidious) onset, and florid presentation.[207]

Acute Phase: Benzodiazepines: If agitation, akathisia, or insomnia is a prominent feature, a benzodiazepine may be prescribed, but the patient should be observed for exacerbations of acute, aggressive behavior.[207]

Maintenance Phase: Maintenance therapy begins upon resolution of the acute episode. Treatment goals in this phase are to maintain or improve the level of functioning and quality of life, and to establish ongoing methods for monitoring compliance and side effects.

Antipsychotic therapy should be continued in schizophrenic patients for at least 12 and possibly as long as 24 months to reduce the risk of relapse. This risk is high (40% to 60%) in those who do not continue therapy after resolution of the initial acute episode.[203] Many, if not most, patients will require lifelong drug therapy. Maintenance therapy with typical antipsychotic drugs is effective but must be balanced against risk of tardive dyskinesia (TD), which

increases with continued drug use. Doses should be reduced during maintenance if the patient is stable, compliant, and not suicidal or violent, and
tapered gradually, every 2 to 4 weeks, over several months. If relapse occurs,
the dose of the typical antipsychotic should be increased to the previous level
or an atypical antipsychotic considered.[203,207] Some patients develop postpsychotic depression requiring antidepressant therapy. Substance abuse issues are
more easily addressed during maintenance.[203]

   Treatment Resistance: Between 15% and 30% of patients have residual
positive symptoms that cannot be controlled with antipsychotic therapy.[210]
Clozapine is available for treatment-resistant patients but requires weekly
hematologic monitoring because of the risk of granulocytopenia (see page
139). There is increasing evidence that the newer atypical antipsychotic drugs,
such as risperidone, olanzapine, and quetiapine, are more effective in refractory patients and have a substantially more favorable side-effect profile than the
typical antipsychotics. Psychiatric referral should be considered for partially or
totally treatment-resistant patients for overall assessment and possible adjunctive therapy with lithium, anticonvulsants, ECT, benzodiazepines, or antidepressants. Full discussion of these approaches is beyond the scope of this
handbook (see references 203 and 207).

Psychopharmacologic Agents

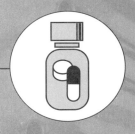

Antidepressants

Antidepressants are effective for depression, for many anxiety disorders, and for some eating disorders. Although the tricyclic antidepressants (TCAs), selective serotonin reuptake inhibitors (SSRIs) (eg, paroxetine, fluoxetine, fluvoxamine, sertraline, citalopram), monoamine oxidase inhibitors (MAOIs), and miscellaneous agents (eg, bupropion, mirtazapine, nefazodone, trazodone, and venlafaxine) are considered comparably effective, their safety and side-effect profiles differ tremendously. Thus, clinicians select an antidepressant drug based on a number of criteria such as tolerability, prior response, concurrent medical conditions, drug interactions, and cost.

TRICYCLIC ANTIDEPRESSANTS

In recent years, the position of TCAs (Tables 40 and 41) as first-line treatment for depression has been supplanted by newer agents that are better tolerated and safer.

Table 40. Overview of oral TCA therapy

Feature	Comments
Mechanism	Inhibit NE (and 5-HT) reuptake acutely but 2- to 4-week delay in clinical response likely due to chronic adaptive changes in neurotransmitter receptor sensitivity or density, signal transduction mechanisms, or changes in gene expression
Pharmacokinetics	Good oral absorption, peak plasma levels in 2 - 6 h; >90% protein-bound, highly lipid-soluble. QD dosing ($t_{1/2}$ 24 h). Extensive metabolism via CYP450; several have active metabolites. Drug interactions common (TCAs inhibit to some extent CYP2D6). Plasma levels of some TCAs (eg, nortriptyline) correlate with efficacy but individualized dosing necessary
Efficacy	Major depression including psychotic (in conjunction with antipsychotic drug) or melancholic subtypes and some anxiety disorders. Other uses: migraine headache, enuresis, chronic pain
Safety	Sedation, dry mouth, orthostatic hypotension, dizziness, constipation. Severe: conduction abnormalities, tachycardia, heart block. Low therapeutic index and therefore highly lethal in overdose
Dosing	Individualize; initiate with low HS dose; ↑ if no response over 7 - 10 days. Wait 2 weeks, if no response, continue to ↑ dose. Clinical response may be delayed for 4 weeks. Use ↓ doses and even slower titration in elderly. Monitor plasma levels at least once and more often in patients experiencing toxic effects or in those suspected of non-compliance

Abbreviations defined in GLOSSARY.

Table 41. Comparative features of oral TCAs[211,212]

Group/drug	Uptake blocking activity NE	Uptake blocking activity 5-HT	Usual dose range (mg/d)	Anti-cholinergic	Sedation	Orthostatic hypotension	Effective plasma level (ng/mL)
TERTIARY AMINES							
Amitriptyline (Elavil®)	++	+++	50 - 300	++++	++++	++	110 - 250[a]
Clomipramine (Anafranil®)	++	+++++	25 - 250	+++	+++	++	80 - 100
Doxepin (Sinequan®)	+	++	25 - 300	+++	+++	++	100 - 200[a]
Imipramine (Tofranil®)	++[b]	+++	30 - 300	++	++	+++	200 - 350[a]
Trimipramine (Surmontil®)	+	+	50 - 300	++	+++	++	180[a]
SECONDARY AMINES							
Amoxapine[c] (Asendin®)	+++	++	50 - 600	+++	++	+	200 - 500
Desipramine (Norpramin®)	++++	++	25 - 300	+	+	+	125 - 300
Nortriptyline (Pamelor®)	++	+++	30 - 100	++	++	+	50 - 150
Protriptyline (Vivactil®)	++++	++	15 - 60	++++	+	+	100 - 200
TETRACYCLIC[d]							
Maprotiline (Ludiomil®)	+++	0/+	50 - 225	++	++	+	200 - 300[a]

+++++ = highest; ++++ = very high; +++ = high; ++ = moderate; + = slight.

Abbreviations defined in GLOSSARY.

[a]Parent plus active metabolite. [b]Via desipramine, the major metabolite. [c]A metabolite of the antipsychotic loxapine; also blocks dopamine receptors. [d]Mirtazapine also is a tetracyclic but differs from TCAs and is reviewed separately.

Information in this table obtained from Physicians' Desk Reference, Facts and Comparisons, or AHFS Drug Information. Please refer to those sources for current and additional prescribing information.

Table 42. Common drug interactions with TCAs[211,213]

Interacting drug	Effect of interaction
Alcohol	↑ Psychomotor impairment
Anticholinergics	TCAs may ↑ anticholinergic effects
Anticoagulants	TCAs may ↓ warfarin metabolism or interfere with protein binding: ↑ therapeutic effect. Monitor PT
Antipsychotics (typical)	Phenothiazines or haloperidol may ↑ TCA levels; TCA also may ↑ antipsychotic levels
Barbiturates	↓ TCA levels; possible ↑ CNS depression
Cimetidine	↑ TCA levels: ↑ anticholinergic effects
Clonidine	TCAs may antagonize antihypertensive effects; may cause hypertensive crisis; avoid concurrent use
Guanethidine	TCAs may antagonize antihypertensive effects; monitor BP closely or avoid concurrent use
Haloperidol	↓ TCA metabolism: ↑ TCA levels and side effects
Levodopa	TCAs may ↓ absorption
MAOIs	Serious serotonin syndrome (see GLOSSARY) possible if TCAs used with or within 7 - 14 days of MAOI. Tertiary TCAs (except clomipramine) may be used with close monitoring
Methylphenidate	↓ TCA metabolism: ↑ TCA levels
Oral contraceptives	↓ TCA metabolism: ↑ TCA levels
Phenothiazines	↓ TCA metabolism: ↑ TCA levels, ↑ anticholinergic side effects. Also, TCA may ↑ phenothiazine level
Phenytoin	TCAs may ↑ phenytoin levels; monitor phenytoin levels. Also, phenytoin may ↓ TCA levels
Quinidine	May ↑ TCA levels by inhibiting metabolism; possible additive effects on cardiac conduction
SSRIs	↓ TCA metabolism: ↑ TCA levels (>100%) and side effects
Sympathomimetic amines[a]	May potentiate arrhythmias, hypertension, tachycardia when used with TCAs

Abbreviations defined in GLOSSARY.

[a]Dextromethorphan, ephedrine, levarterenol, mephentermine, methylphenidate, phenylephrine, phenylpropanolamine, pseudoephedrine.

Information in this table obtained from *Physicians' Desk Reference*, *Facts and Comparisons*, or *AHFS Drug Information*. Please refer to those sources for current and additional prescribing information.

Efficacy

All TCAs are effective for the treatment of major depression and its sub-types (eg, melancholia) and some anxiety disorders. Clomipramine carries Food and Drug Administration (FDA)-approved labeling only for the treatment of obsessive-compulsive disorder (OCD).[211]

Drug Interactions

Drug interactions with TCAs are caused through interference with hepatic metabolism or potentiation of central nervous system (CNS) side effects (Table 42). The interaction with MAOIs is of special importance, although this combination is not routinely used in the primary care setting. Under expert medical supervision, the combination of a TCA (but not clomipramine, because of its serotonergic properties) and an MAOI can be therapeutically useful and, with appropriate monitoring, may be safe.

Safety

Because they interact with a variety of CNS receptors (Table 43), TCAs cause a number of clinically important side effects that are troublesome enough in younger, otherwise healthy individuals but that can be severe, debilitating, and treatment-limiting in the elderly or patients with underlying medical conditions (especially cardiac disease).[214,215]

For example, the elderly are especially sensitive to side effects related to interactions with cholinergic and α-adrenergic receptors; falls and bone injuries are more common in this population.[216] Dose-related toxic psychosis (confusion, delirium) occurs at lower plasma levels in the elderly than in younger patients.[214]

Table 43. Common side effects of TCAs

Receptor	Common examples
Anticholinergic	Dry mouth, constipation, blurry vision, urinary retention, cognitive impairment in the elderly
Antihistaminic	Sedation, weight gain
Serotonergic	Sexual dysfunction
α-Adrenergic	Orthostatic hypotension, dizziness

Abbreviations defined in GLOSSARY.

Information in this table obtained from *Physicians' Desk Reference, Facts and Comparisons,* or *AHFS Drug Information.* Please refer to those sources for current and additional prescribing information.

Tolerance may develop to some TCA side effects, but low starting doses and gradual upward titration can minimize these effects early on. Other common side effects include confusion, headache, rash, nausea, and vomiting.

Photosensitivity may occur. Although not all products are rated, most TCAs are rated Pregnancy Category C (see GLOSSARY; see also DRUG USE IN PREGNANCY/LACTATION, page 162) and are excreted in breast milk in low concentrations; maprotiline is excreted in breast milk at levels comparable to plasma.

Warnings/Precautions

In usual doses, TCAs may induce angina and cause arrhythmias, conduction abnormalities, or tachycardia. Thus, use TCAs cautiously and with electrocardiographic (ECG) monitoring in patients with cardiovascular diseases or hyperthyroidism, and avoid use in the immediate postmyocardial infarction (MI) period. TCAs have a narrow therapeutic index; ingestion of as little as 1 or 2 weeks' worth of medication can cause serious toxicity and may be fatal. Patients with suicidal thoughts, plans, or attempts should not be given large quantities of TCAs. In TCA overdose, cardiac toxicity is caused by strong anticholinergic effects and a quinidine-like effect that causes heart block, depressed contractility, severe arrhythmias, cardiac arrest, and sudden death.

TCAs can lower the seizure threshold and may cause seizures in patients with or without a prior history; this effect may be dose related. Maprotiline is contraindicated in patients with seizure disorders and should be administered in divided doses when used at the upper dose range. Because of their strong anticholinergic effects, use TCAs cautiously in patients with urinary retention or angle-closure glaucoma. Bone marrow depression and hepatitis have been reported; baseline and periodic white blood cell (WBC) and liver function test (LFT) monitoring may be needed. Patients with schizophrenia or bipolar disorders may experience development or exaggeration of psychosis or mania/hypomania, respectively, while on TCA therapy.

Dosing Guidelines

Individualize dose and titration (refer to prescribing information of specific products for more information). In general, initiate therapy with a single bedtime (HS) dose at the lower end of the dosage range (see Table 41) and titrate upward gradually over 1 to 2 weeks if a response does not occur. Maintain this dose for an additional 2 weeks and then increase further if tolerated. A full therapeutic response may require 2 to 4 weeks to develop. The elderly and those with severe renal or hepatic impairment usually require lower starting doses and more gradual titration to minimize toxicity. Therapeutic plasma levels are probably the same as in younger adults. Abrupt discontinuation may cause a rebound in cholinergic side effects; reduce doses gradually, by 25 to 50 mg every 3 to 7 days.

SELECTIVE SEROTONIN REUPTAKE INHIBITORS

SSRIs available in the US for the treatment of depression and several anxiety disorders (eg, OCD, panic disorder [PD]) include fluoxetine, paroxetine, and sertraline; fluvoxamine currently is aproved by the FDA only for treatment of OCD and citalopram is approved only for depression (Tables 44 and 45). Paroxetine is the only SSRI approved for social anxiety disorder.

Table 44. Overview of SSRI therapy

Feature	Comments
Mechanism	Potent, selective inhibition of 5-HT reuptake causes ↑ 5-HT activity in synapse.[217] Weak effects on NE and DA reuptake, minimal effects on cholinergic, histaminic, GABA, and α- or β-adrenergic receptors
Pharmacokinetics	Well absorbed orally, peak levels in 6 h (see Table 46); no clinically important effect of food on absorption.[218] Extensive hepatic metabolism via CYP450. Half-life and presence of pharmacologically active metabolites are pharmacokinetic distinctions. Drug interactions potentially common. No correlation between efficacy and plasma levels
Efficacy	First-line treatment for depression (with or without anxious features) and many anxiety disorders (OCD, PD, social anxiety disorder)
Safety	Transient dizziness, drowsiness, tremor, sweating, headache, dry mouth, diarrhea, nausea, vomiting, sexual dysfunction, "jitteriness" reported. Much safer than TCAs in overdose. Abrupt cessation can result in transient discontinuation symptoms ("electrical sensations" in upper extremities, dizziness, malaise)
Dosing	QD dosing; ↑ dose gradually if needed after 2 - 3 weeks (longer for fluoxetine). Full response in 4 - 6 weeks; ↓ starting doses in elderly, patients with renal or hepatic dysfunction, or marked anxiety

Abbreviations defined in GLOSSARY.

Table 45. Comparative features of SSRIs[212,219]

| Drug | Uptake blocking activity | | | Usual dose range (mg/d) | Anticholinergic | Sedation | Orthostatic hypotension | Effective plasma level (ng/mL) |
	DA	NE	5-HT					
Paroxetine (Paxil®)	0	0/+	+++++	20 - 50	0/+	0/+	0	NR
Fluoxetine (Prozac®)	0	0/+	+++++	20 - 60	0	0/+	0	NR
Sertraline (Zoloft®)	0/+	0/+	+++++	50 - 200	0	0/+	0	NR
Fluvoxamine (Luvox®)	0	0/+	++++	50 - 300	0	0/+	0	NR
Citalopram (Celexa®)	0	0	+++++	20 - 40	0	0/+	0	NR

+++++ = highest; ++++ = very high; +++ = high; ++ = moderate; + = slight; 0 = none. NR = not relevant to clinical response; other abbreviations defined in GLOSSARY.

Information in this table obtained from *Physicians' Desk Reference, Facts and Comparisons,* or *AHFS Drug Information.* Please refer to those sources for current and additional prescribing information.

Table 46. Comparative pharmacokinetic features of SSRIs[218,219]

Drug	T_{max} (h)	$T_{1/2}$	% Protein binding	Time to reach steady-state (d)	Elimination route
Paroxetine	3 - 8	21 h	93 - 95	7 - 10	64% renal; 36% hepatic
Fluoxetine	6 - 8	4 - 6 d	95	28 - 35	Hepatic
norfluoxetine[a]	—	4 - 16 d	—	—	—
Sertraline	4 - 9	26 h	98	7 - 10	40% - 45% renal; 40% - 45% hepatic
desmethylsertraline[a]	—	2 - 4 d	—	—	—
Fluvoxamine	4 - 8	14 - 16 h	77 - 80	7 - 10	Renal
Citalopram	2 - 4	33 h	80	7 - 10	Hepatic
demethylcitalopram[a]	—	2 d	—	—	—
didemethylcitalopram[a]	—	4 d	—	—	—

Abbreviations defined in GLOSSARY.

[a]Active metabolite.

Information in this table obtained from *Physicians' Desk Reference, Facts and Comparisons,* or *AHFS Drug Information.* Please refer to those sources for current and additional prescribing information.

Efficacy

SSRIs are a proven effective first-line treatment for depression and are as effective as other antidepressants.[216,220-225] SSRIs also are an established treatment for many anxiety disorders (eg, PD, OCD, and social anxiety disorders).[26] SSRIs are preferred for many patients with comorbid medical conditions (see Table 17).

Drug Interactions

Drug interactions with SSRIs are caused by displacement from protein binding sites or inhibition of hepatic CYP450 isoenzymes (Table 47). Each of the SSRIs inhibits different CYP enzyme systems to various degrees, indicating that specific interactions are not a class effect. Nonetheless, clinicians should be alert to the possibility of an interaction between an SSRI and any drug that is extensively metabolized by CYP isoenzymes (see comprehensive review of this topic in reference 213). Concurrent use of an SSRI and an MAOI is absolutely contraindicated; patients who start MAOI therapy within 14 days of discontinuing an SSRI (up to 5 weeks with long-acting fluoxetine) may develop a serious and possibly fatal reaction called the "serotonin syndrome" (see GLOSSARY).

Psychopharmacologic Agents

Table 47. Common drug interactions with SSRIs[213,226]

Interacting drug	Effect of interaction
Anticoagulants	Displacement of warfarin from protein-binding sites may ↑ PT; monitor PT
Atypical antipsychotics	↑ Clozapine levels
β-Blockers	↑ Plasma levels
Benzodiazepines[a]	↓ Benzodiazepine clearance: ↑ levels
Carbamazepine	↑ Carbamazepine levels may cause toxicity (fluoxetine, fluvoxamine, sertraline)
Haloperidol	↓ Haloperidol metabolism: ↑ levels (fluvoxamine)
Lithium	Lithium may ↑ serotonergic effects of SSRIs
MAOIs	Serious serotonin syndrome (see GLOSSARY) possible when SSRIs used with or within 14[b] days of MAOI therapy
Nonsedating antihistamines (astemizole)	Avoid concurrent use of drugs that inhibit CYP3A4
Phenobarbital, phenytoin	Fluoxetine may ↑ anticonvulsant levels; anticonvulsants also ↓ paroxetine $t_{1/2}$
TCAs	↓ TCA metabolism: ↑ TCA levels and side effects
Theophylline	↓ Theophylline clearance (fluvoxamine), ↑ levels; ↓ theophylline dose, monitor levels
Trazodone	Paroxetine may ↓ trazodone metabolism: ↑ side effects (serotonin syndrome)
Type 1C antiarrhythmics (encainide, flecainide)	↑ Antiarrhythmic levels; avoid concurrent use

Abbreviations defined in GLOSSARY.

[a]Only benzodiazepines metabolized by oxidation are affected (see Table 68).

[b]Washout period of several weeks may be needed for SSRIs with long $t_{1/2}$ (eg, fluoxetine).

Information in this table obtained from *Physicians' Desk Reference, Facts and Comparisons,* or *AHFS Drug Information.* Please refer to those sources for current and additional prescribing information.

Safety

An important advantage of SSRIs is their excellent safety and tolerability profile. They lack anticholinergic- and adrenergic-mediated side effects of TCAs (eg, orthostasis, cardiac conduction changes, blurry vision, dry mouth, etc). They are far safer than TCAs in acute overdose situations and have little effect on ECG parameters or blood pressure (BP).[214] Fatal and nonfatal overdoses of citalopram have been associated with prolonged QT intervals, sinus tachycardia, and repolarization changes.[227,228]

Common, transient, SSRI side effects include dizziness, drowsiness, tremor, sweating, headache, dry mouth, diarrhea, nausea, and vomiting (tolerance usually develops to nausea). SSRIs have similar overall safety profiles. However, fluoxetine may cause treatment-emergent anxiety, nervousness, and insomnia; paroxetine may cause somnolence; and sertraline may cause diarrhea.[220] In the first few weeks after initiation of therapy, up to 16% of patients may experience a "jitteriness" or "activation" syndrome, consisting of anxiety, restlessness, nervousness, insomnia, and gastrointestinal (GI) symptoms; this syndrome may be more common with fluoxetine. If not advised of this and counseled that the syndrome will resolve with time, patients may discontinue treatment. A brief course of benzodiazepine therapy (eg, alprazolam or clonazepam) during the SSRI initiation period may reduce the duration and severity of symptoms,[229] although certainly the more prudent approach would be to use low SSRI doses and increase slowly.

Sexual dysfunction occurs with all SSRIs to a greater degree than with TCAs. True incidence figures are difficult to ascertain because sexual problems are typically underreported, but estimates as high as 25% to 50% of at least mild symptoms have been suggested. Complaints include decreased libido, arousal, and duration and intensity of orgasm.[230] Men complain of impotence and a decreased ability to ejaculate. Rare cases of female sexual hyperstimulation have been reported.[231,232] Short-term weight loss can occur and may be more common with fluoxetine. Transient, asymptomatic LFT increases may occur in the first several weeks of sertraline therapy; these normalize when the drug is discontinued. SSRIs are rated Pregnancy Category C (see GLOSSARY; see also DRUG USE IN PREGNANCY/LACTATION, page 162). They should be used cautiously in nursing mothers because, like all antidepressants, SSRIs are excreted in breast milk.[233] However, individual SSRIs are eliminated in breast milk to varying degrees (see Table 101).

Warnings/Precautions

Patients treated with fluoxetine may develop a rash with leukocytosis, fever, edema, respiratory distress, lymphadenopathy, proteinuria, and mildly elevated LFTs. A systemic illness resembling vasculitis is rare but has developed in patients with the rash; dyspnea may be the first and only symptom. Fluoxetine should be discontinued if a rash appears.

Fluoxetine may cause hypoglycemia; the dose of insulin or sulfonylurea may require adjustment. SSRIs should be used carefully in patients with seizure disorders.

Dosing Guidelines

Fluoxetine: Usual starting dose for depression: 20 mg once daily (QD) in the morning. As with all antidepressants, clinical response may be delayed for a few to several weeks. If needed, increase gradually to a maximum of 80 mg/d. Usual starting dose for OCD: 20 mg QD in the morning for 2 weeks; increase to 40 mg QD if necessary. Usual range is 40 to 60 mg/d, but some patients may require up to 80 mg/d (maximum). Usual starting dose for bulimia nervosa (BN): 60 mg/d. For all indications, use a lower dose (10 mg) or a less frequent administration schedule in the elderly or patients with renal or hepatic dysfunction. A long elimination half-life and active metabolite contribute to a prolonged duration of drug effects upon dosage adjustment or termination of therapy.

Fluvoxamine: Usual starting dose for OCD: 50 mg HS; increase by 50 mg/d every 4 to 7 days if needed to a maximum of 300 mg/d. When the total dose of this short half-life drug is higher than 100 mg/d, divide into two equal doses to minimize side effects; if unequal, give the larger dose HS. Use lower initial doses in the elderly or patients with hepatic impairment.

Paroxetine: Usual starting dose for depression: 20 mg QD in the morning. If response is inadequate after 2 to 3 weeks, increase weekly by 10 mg/d to a maximum of 50 mg/d. Use a lower initial dose (10 mg QD) in the elderly and renally or hepatically impaired patients; increase to a maximum of 40 mg/d as needed. Usual starting dose for PD: 10 mg QD in the morning; increase weekly by 10 mg/d to a target dose of 40 mg/d. The maximum dose is 60 mg/d. Usual starting dose for OCD: 20 mg QD in the morning; increase not more than weekly by 10 mg/d to 60 mg/d (maximum). Usual starting dose for social anxiety disorder: 20 mg QD in the morning. If response is inadequate, increase not more than weekly by 10 mg/d to 60 mg/d (maximum).

Sertraline: Usual starting dose: 50 mg QD (morning or evening); if response is inadequate after 1 week or more, increase gradually to a maximum of 200 mg/d. Most patients require 100 to 150 mg/d. In the elderly or in patients with hepatic or renal impairment, begin therapy with 25 mg QD in the morning.

Citalopram: Usual starting dose: 20 mg QD (morning or evening); increase dose to 40 mg/d after 1 week. The starting dose in elderly patients or patients with hepatic impairment is 20 mg/d, increasing to 40 mg/d in nonresponding patients.

When stopping therapy with any SSRI, taper gradually to minimize discontinuation symptoms (eg, anxiety, dizziness, headache, flu-like symptoms, paresthesias) that could occur with abrupt discontinuation.[234] Educate patients about the often transient nature of these side effects and advise them not to stop therapy without a consultation. Discontinuation symptoms for SSRIs with shorter elimination half-lives (eg, paroxetine, fluvoxamine, sertraline) generally persist for 1 to 2 weeks after treatment cessation. Fluoxetine may cause discontinuation symptoms beginning up to 25 days after stopping therapy because of its longer elimination half-life[235] (see Table 46); these symptoms may persist for up to 56 days.

MONOAMINE OXIDASE INHIBITORS

For nearly 40 years, MAOIs have provided an effective treatment for depression. Two MAOIs are widely available in the US: phenelzine (Nardil®) and tranylcypromine (Parnate®) (Table 48); isocarboxazid (Marplan®) is available only on a very limited basis. However, serious safety issues that require compliance with the prescribed regimen and strict adherence to dietary restrictions have relegated these drugs to third-line status.

Table 48. Overview of MAOI therapy

Feature	Comments
Mechanism	Irreversible, nonselective inhibition of monoamine oxidase → ↑ levels of epinephrine, NE, 5-HT
Pharmacokinetics	Limited data; good oral absorption. Efficacy not correlated with plasma levels. Drug/food interactions common
Efficacy	Third-line treatment for uncomplicated major depression; useful for geriatric, atypical, or bipolar depression and social anxiety disorder
Safety	Orthostatic hypotension, dizziness, headache, dry mouth, insomnia, nausea, constipation or diarrhea, anorexia or weight gain. Hypertensive crisis if tyramine-containing foods or sympathomimetic drugs ingested (see Tables 49, 50)
Dosing	Phenelzine 15 mg TID; ↑ to 60 - 90 mg/d as tolerated. Response may be delayed ≥4 weeks. ↓ Dose gradually over several weeks when discontinuation is desired. Tranylcypromine 30 mg/d (divided); if no response in 2 weeks, ↑ by 10 mg/d (60 mg/d maximum) every 1 - 2 weeks

Abbreviations defined in GLOSSARY.

Efficacy

Phenelzine and tranylcypromine are equally effective[236] although the onset of clinical activity may be faster with tranylcypromine (10 days) than with phenelzine (3 to 4 weeks) because the former may have amphetamine-like properties; clinical effects continue for days (tranylcypromine) to weeks (phenelzine) after therapy is discontinued. MAOIs are rarely a first-line treatment for depression because of important safety issues (ie, hypertensive crisis, serotonin syndrome, sexual dysfunction); however, they are a reasonable alternative for bipolar depression, depressed patients with atypical features, social anxiety disorder, or for patients unresponsive to other antidepressants.[236-238]

Drug/Food Interactions

Ingestion of tyramine-containing foods (Table 49) or sympathomimetic amines (eg, over-the-counter [OTC] cough/cold or allergy products or appetite suppressants) may induce hypertensive crisis. Other interactions are listed in Table 50.

Table 49. Tyramine-containing foods (adapted from reference 239, with permission).
© Copyright 1996, Physicians Postgraduate Press.

Restriction	Sample foods
Avoid	Aged cheeses; aged or cured meats (eg, salami, pastrami, dry or summer sausage, mortadella); spoiled or improperly stored meats, poultry, or fish; broad (fava) beans; Marmite yeast extract; sauerkraut; soy sauce/condiments; tap beer
Use in moderation	Red or white wine (8 ounces/d), domestic bottled or canned beer (2 bottles or cans/d) (including nonalcoholic beer)[a]
Allowed	Avocados; banana pulp; beef/chicken bouillon; chocolate; fresh or mild cheese or milk products (eg, cottage cheese, ricotta, cream cheese); fresh meat, fish, poultry; peanuts; soy milk; properly stored fresh smoked or pickled fish (eg, herring)

[a]Some authorities advocate elimination of all beer and red wine because tyramine content is variable between brands.

Safety

Common side effects include orthostatic hypotension, dizziness, headache, dry mouth, hypomania in bipolar patients (in those using higher doses or on long-term treatment), insomnia or hypersomnia, nausea, constipation or diarrhea, peripheral edema, skin rash, and anorexia or weight gain. Safe use during pregnancy or in nursing mothers has not been established (see also DRUG USE IN PREGNANCY/LACTATION, page 162).

Warnings/Precautions

MAOIs are contraindicated in patients with pheochromocytoma, liver disease or abnormal LFTs, severe renal impairment, cerebrovascular disease, history of headaches, cardiovascular disease, congestive heart failure (CHF), or hypertension, and in patients older than 60 years who may have damaged or sclerotic cerebral vessels.

Table 50. Common drug interactions with MAOIs[236]

Interacting drug	Effect of interaction
β-Blockers	Bradycardia possible during concurrent use
Antidiabetic agents	May ↑ hypoglycemic response or delay recovery from hypoglycemia
Barbiturates	↑ CNS depression
Bupropion	↑ Acute bupropion toxicity (phenelzine, animal data). Concurrent use contraindicated; wait ≥14 d after stopping MAOI before starting bupropion
Carbamazepine	Concurrent use contraindicated; allow ≥14 d between discontinuation of MAOI and initiation of carbamazepine
L-Tryptophan[a]	Hyperthermia, hyperventilation, confusion, delirium, agitation, hypomania possible; avoid concurrent use
Meperidine	Serotonin syndrome (see GLOSSARY) possible, severe fever, coma, rigidity, excitation, hypertension (may be fatal); use other narcotic analgesics
Nefazodone	Although not directly evaluated, serotonin syndrome (see GLOSSARY) possible when nefazodone used within 14 days of stopping MAOI. Allow 7 days between stopping nefazodone and starting MAOI
Sympathomimetic amines[b]	Hypertensive crisis possible; may be fatal (see Warnings/ Precautions, page 89)
TCAs, SSRIs	Serious serotonin syndrome (see GLOSSARY) possible when antidepressants used with or within 14[c] days of an MAOI. Tertiary TCAs (except clomipramine) may be acceptable with close monitoring. Concurrent use of SSRIs contraindicated
Trazodone	Serotonin syndrome (see GLOSSARY) possible when trazodone used within 14 days of stopping MAOI. May be dose related (seen at doses ≥150 mg/d) but combination generally not recommended. Allow 7 days between stopping trazodone and starting MAOI

Abbreviations defined in GLOSSARY.

[a]Not available as a drug in the US other than in some herbal preparations.

[b]Dextromethorphan, ephedrine, levarterenol, mephentermine, methylphenidate, phenylephrine, phenylpropanolamine, pseudoephedrine.

[c]Washout period of several weeks may be needed for SSRIs with long $t_{1/2}$ (eg, fluoxetine).

Information in this table obtained from Physicians' Desk Reference, Facts and Comparisons, or AHFS Drug Information. Please refer to those sources for current and additional prescribing information.

Hypertensive crisis (also called the "cheese effect"), sometimes fatal, can occur within hours after a patient has ingested a banned food or drug substance (Tables 48 and 49). The first symptom may be severe headache, neck stiffness, or palpitations followed by nausea, vomiting, sweating, dilated pupils, and constricting chest pain with tachycardia or bradycardia. Patients should be instructed to seek emergency medical attention if these symptoms develop. Discontinue MAOI therapy immediately if these signs and symptoms develop, and initiate proper cardiovascular treatment and supportive care immediately if hypertension is severe. Treatments include administration of an α_1-blocker such as phentolamine or a calcium channel blocker (eg, nifedipine 10 mg orally).

Dosing Guidelines

Phenelzine: Initial dose: 15 mg three times daily (TID); increase to 60 to 90 mg/d as tolerated. Clinical response may not be evident for 4 weeks or more at this dosage level. Reduce dose gradually over several weeks.

Tranylcypromine: Usual dose: 30 mg/d (divided). If no improvement within 2 weeks, increase by 10 mg/d every 1 to 2 weeks to a maximum of 60 mg/d. Withdrawal should be gradual. Dietary counseling and monitoring are recommended.

MISCELLANEOUS ANTIDEPRESSANTS

The miscellaneous antidepressants (Table 51) bupropion (Table 52), mirtazapine (Table 54), nefazodone (Table 56), trazodone (Table 58), and venlafaxine (Table 60) are structurally dissimilar to TCAs, SSRIs, or MAOIs. Each is discussed briefly in the next sections.

Table 51. Comparative features of miscellaneous oral antidepressants[212]

Drug	Uptake blocking activity			Usual dose range (mg/d)	Anticholinergic	Sedation	Orthostatic hypotension
	DA	NE	5-HT				
Bupropion (Wellbutrin®)	+	0/+	0/+	200 - 450	0	0/+	+
Mirtazapine (Remeron™)	0	+	0	15 - 45	0	++++	0
Nefazodone (Serzone®)	0	+	++	200 - 600	0	++	+
Trazodone (Desyrel®)	0	0	++	150 - 600	0	+++	++
Venlafaxine (Effexor®, Effexor® XR)	0	++	+++	75 - 375	0	0	0

+++++ = highest; ++++ = very high; +++ = high; ++ = moderate; + = slight; 0 = none; other abbreviations defined in GLOSSARY.

Information in this table obtained from *Physicians' Desk Reference, Facts and Comparisons*, or *AHFS Drug Information*. Please refer to those sources for current and additional prescribing information.

BUPROPION

Bupropion (Wellbutrin®) is available as an immediate-release and a new sustained-release product (see NICOTINE ABUSE AND DEPENDENCE, page 52).

Table 52. Overview of bupropion therapy

Feature	Comments
Mechanism	Exact mechanism not fully known; weakly blocks NE, DA, and 5-HT reuptake; mild DA agonist. Active metabolite (hydroxy-bupropion) selectively blocks NE but not 5-HT reuptake[240]
Pharmacokinetics	Peak levels in 2 h (3 h for sustained-release); $t_{1/2}$ 14 h (immediate-release) to 21 h (sustained-release), 80% to 85% protein bound. Several active metabolites. Hepatic or renal disease or CHF may alter metabolism or elimination. No consistent relation between efficacy and plasma levels, but trough levels 20 - 40 ng/mL may correlate with efficacy
Efficacy	Comparable to TCAs, SSRIs for depression but not first-line (titration/seizure issues). Also social anxiety disorder, bipolar depression
Safety	Dry mouth, nausea; nonsedating but troublesome CNS stimulation. Rare orthostatic hypotension. May ↑ or ↓ sexual function. Seizures are serious but low risk, limited to the immediate-release formulation, and seen primarily in patients with BN
Dosing	Immediate-release: 100 mg BID, ↑ to 100 mg TID after 3 days, wait several weeks before ↑ to 150 mg TID. Maximum 450 mg/d, 150 mg/dose. Sustained-release: 150 mg QD, ↑ to 150 mg BID after 4 days; maximum dose 200 mg BID. Always ↑ slowly to ↓ seizure risk and stimulation. ↓ Dose in renal or hepatic disease

Abbreviations defined in GLOSSARY.

Efficacy

Bupropion is comparable in efficacy to TCAs and SSRIs but is not usually a first-line antidepressant because of certain safety issues (eg, seizures) with the immediate-release formulation.[241] Bupropion has traditionally been used for patients resistant to or intolerant of other antidepressants or for those with atypical depression because of its activating side effects.[216] Because it generally lacks adverse effects on sexual function, bupropion may be considered an alternative for patients experiencing sexual dysfunction with other types of antidepressant therapy.[230] Because sexual stimulation has been reported with bupropion,[230] this drug could be added to an antidepressant regimen to reduce sexual dysfunction. Bupropion has been reported to be effective in social anxiety disorder and bipolar illness but is not to be used for BN (see Warnings/Precautions) or PD. There is one report of its use in depressed, post-MI patients.[242]

Drug Interactions

Bupropion may induce its own metabolism as well as the metabolism of other drugs (Table 53).

Table 53. Common drug interactions with bupropion[241]

Interacting drug	Effect of interaction
Alcohol	May ↓ seizure threshold; limit or avoid alcohol use
Carbamazepine	Carbamazepine may ↓ bupropion levels
Levodopa	↑ Levodopa side effects; ↓ levodopa dose
Lithium	May ↑ seizure risk
MAOIs	↑ Acute bupropion toxicity (phenelzine, animal data). Concurrent use contraindicated; wait ≥14 d after stopping MAOI before starting bupropion
Valproic acid	Bupropion may ↑ valproic acid levels

Abbreviations defined in GLOSSARY.

Information in this table obtained from *Physicians' Desk Reference, Facts and Comparisons,* or *AHFS Drug Information.* Please refer to those sources for current and additional prescribing information.

Safety

Bupropion has a relatively mild side-effect profile as compared with TCAs. It is not sedating, it lacks strong anticholinergic side effects, and has a safer cardiac profile than TCAs (ie, insignificant ECG changes). Dry mouth and nausea are common early in treatment, but orthostatic hypotension is rare. Sexual dysfunction is infrequent as compared with other antidepressants (eg, SSRIs); paradoxically, improvement or overstimulation of sexual function also has been reported.[230,243] Because it has mild dopaminergic activity, bupropion may cause CNS stimulation (eg, restlessness, agitation, insomnia) that either may require temporary ancillary treatment (ie, sedative/hypnotic) or may cause discontinuation of therapy. This side effect may be beneficial in withdrawn, depressed individuals, however.[243] Weight loss may be greater than with other antidepressants. Bupropion is rated Pregnancy Category B (see GLOSSARY; see also DRUG USE IN PREGNANCY/LACTATION, page 162); assess risks before prescribing to nursing mothers.

Warnings/Precautions

Bupropion is contraindicated in seizure disorder, current or past diagnosis of BN or anorexia nervosa (AN), and in persons currently using an MAOI or in those who stopped MAOI therapy fewer than 14 days earlier. The risk of seizures with immediate-release bupropion is approximately 0.4% (4/1000) at a dose of 450 mg/d. Seizures are more common with high total daily doses (>450 mg/d) or high single doses (>150 mg) and in those with predisposing factors (eg, head trauma, CNS tumor), and can occur at any time during the course of therapy. Use bupropion cautiously in patients with concurrently administered antipsychotics or in abrupt benzodiazepine or alcohol withdrawal, which lowers the seizure threshold (see Dosing Guidelines below).[241] Seizure occurs in about one third of overdose cases; fatalities are due to multiple seizures, bradycardia, and cardiac arrest.

Dosing Guidelines

Usual starting dose (immediate release): 100 mg twice daily (BID); increase to 100 mg TID after 3 days. Maintain this dosage for several weeks to assess full clinical response before increasing to the maximum recommended dose of 150 mg TID (450 mg/d). Usual starting dose (sustained-release): 150 mg QD, increase to 150 mg BID after 4 days; maximum dose 200 mg BID. Use lower doses in patients with renal or hepatic disease to avoid accumulation of bupropion or its active metabolites. Seizure risk can be reduced by using the sustained-release formulation or by limiting the total daily immediate-release dose to 450 mg, single doses to 150 mg, and by adhering to a TID or QID dosing schedule to avoid high peak levels. Increase bupropion doses gradually and by not more than 100 mg/d every 3 days to reduce the risk of seizure and of stimulatory side effects. Avoid HS administration to minimize insomnia; lower the dose of bupropion or use an intermediate- to long-acting benzodiazepine during the first week of therapy if insomnia is bothersome.

MIRTAZAPINE

Table 54. Overview of mirtazapine therapy

Feature	Comments
Mechanism	Blocks α_2 (inhibitory) and specific 5-HT receptors (5-HT$_2$, 5-HT$_3$) $\rightarrow \uparrow$ 5-HT and NE transmission. Weakly inhibits NE reuptake; no effect on DA uptake or receptors. Also a potent H$_1$-blocker, weak inhibitory effects on NE reuptake, weak α_1-receptor antagonism, and moderate activity at cholinergic receptors[244]
Pharmacokinetics	Complete oral absorption unaffected by food. Peak levels in 2 h, 85% protein bound. Highly metabolized via CYP450; QD dosing (t$_{1/2} \geq$21 h). Clearance $\downarrow$ in elderly and in hepatic or renal disease. No therapeutic plasma range; no known drug interactions
Efficacy	Comparable to TCAs or trazodone for depression; limited data in other disorders
Safety	Significant sedation, $\uparrow$ appetite, weight gain, dizziness. Better tolerated than TCAs. Severe: agranulocytosis possible but rare
Dosing	15 mg HS; $\uparrow$ every 1 - 2 weeks to 45 mg HS maximum. Higher doses used in Europe. $\downarrow$ Dose in elderly and renal or hepatic impairment

Abbreviations defined in GLOSSARY.

Efficacy

Mirtazapine (Remeron™) is as effective as TCAs (eg, doxepin, amitriptyline, clomipramine) and trazodone for treatment of depression. Comparative data with SSRIs are not yet available. Efficacy data for other psychiatric indications (eg, anxiety disorders) are limited.[244]

Drug Interactions

In vitro, mirtazapine is a less potent inhibitor of CYP450 isoenzymes than are SSRIs, but in vivo clinical data are sparse. Use of mirtazapine with CNS depressants (eg, alcohol, diazepam) may cause additive psychomotor impairment due to pharmacodynamic interactions[244] (Table 55).

Table 55. Common drug interactions with mirtazapine[245]

Interacting drug	Effect of interaction
Alcohol	↑ Psychomotor impairment
Diazepam	↑ Psychomotor impairment
MAOIs	Avoid concurrent use; do not administer within 14 days of each other

Abbreviations defined in GLOSSARY.

Information in this table obtained from *Physicians' Desk Reference, Facts and Comparisons,* or *AHFS Drug Information.* Please refer to those sources for current and additional prescribing information.

Safety

Mirtazapine appears to be better tolerated than TCAs, but safety data continue to emerge with this new drug as more experience is gained. Comparative frequency data with other antidepressants are limited.[244] Sedation (>50%), increased appetite (17%), weight gain, and dizziness are prominent side effects; tolerance may develop to the former. In controlled trials, overall frequencies of anticholinergic, serotonin-related (eg, nausea, vomiting, agitation, headache, diarrhea), antihistaminic, sexual dysfunction, and cardiac effects were lower than with TCAs. Extrapyramidal side effects (EPS) and orthostatic hypotension are uncommon. In overdose situations, somnolence, disorientation, and tachycardia were the primary symptoms; seizures or cardiac conduction abnormalities common to TCAs were not noted.[244] Mirtazapine is rated Pregnancy Category C (see GLOSSARY; see also DRUG USE IN PREGNANCY/LACTATION, page 162); no data are available regarding its excretion in breast milk.

Warnings/Precautions

Agranulocytosis and asymptomatic severe neutropenia occurred in premarketing clinical trials (3 of nearly 2800 patients). Recovery was complete after discontinuation of the drug. Although agranulocytosis has not been reported in postmarketing surveillance studies in the Netherlands,[245] advise patients to report sore throat, fever, flu-like illness, or other signs of infection. If these signs are present, check WBC count and immediately stop mirtazapine therapy if agranulocytosis is suspected.

Dosing Guidelines

Usual starting dose: 15 mg HS; increase at 1- to 2-week intervals to a maximum of 45 mg HS. As with other antidepressants, clinical response may be delayed for several weeks. Reduce the dose of mirtazapine in the elderly and those with moderate to severe renal impairment.

NEFAZODONE

Table 56. Overview of nefazodone therapy

Feature	Comments
Mechanism	↑ 5-HT neurotransmission via potent antagonism of 5-HT_{2A} receptors. Blocks 5-HT (mild) and NE (weak) reuptake. α_1-Receptor antagonist with low affinity for cholinergic, α_2-adrenergic, DA, and histamine receptors[246]
Pharmacokinetics	Rapid oral absorption (peak levels in 1 h) but is delayed with concurrent food intake, BID dosing ($t_{1/2}$ <4 h); >99% protein bound. Highly metabolized by CYP3A4; two active metabolites. Hepatic clearance ↓ in elderly. Clinically important drug interactions
Efficacy	Major depression; not widely studied for other indications
Safety	Nausea, somnolence, dry mouth, dizziness, constipation, blurry vision. ↓ Activating effects as compared with SSRIs. Sexual dysfunction or priapism are not problems
Dosing	Manufacturer recommends 100 mg BID (50 mg BID in elderly) but we recommend 50 mg BID (50 mg QD in elderly); ↑ by 50 - 100 mg/d after 1 week as tolerated. Minimal effective dose: 300 mg QD. No dosage adjustments for patients with renal impairment

Abbreviations defined in GLOSSARY.

Efficacy

Nefazodone (Serzone®) is effective for the treatment of depression and is comparable in efficacy to TCAs and SSRIs.[246] It has not yet been widely studied for other indications.

Drug Interactions

Clinically important drug interactions with nefazodone are primarily related to its high affinity for and blockade of CYP3A4 isoenzymes (Table 57), although interactions with highly protein-bound drugs can occur.[213,246]

Safety

Nefazodone is generally well tolerated; nausea, somnolence, dry mouth, dizziness, constipation, and blurry vision are common (≥5% incidence). Activating side effects (eg, agitation, tremor, insomnia, nervousness) are less common than with SSRIs. Sexual dysfunction, priapism, and significant weight gain are uncommon with this drug. Nefazodone usually does not disrupt normal sleep (ie, increase rapid eye movement [REM] sleep latency); this feature may be beneficial in some depressed patients.[246] Visual trails have been reported.

Table 57. Common drug interactions with nefazodone[213,246]

Interacting drug	Effect of interaction
Benzodiazepines	Nefazodone ↓ alprazolam, triazolam clearance: ↑ levels, ↑ psychomotor impairment. ↓ Triazolam dose if used concurrently or avoid altogether. No interaction with lorazepam
Carbamazepine	↑ Carbamazepine levels: ↑ toxicity
Cisapride	Concurrent use absolutely contraindicated; ↑ risk of fatal ventricular arrhythmias
Digoxin	↑ Digoxin levels; monitor
Haloperidol	↓ Haloperidol clearance but no ↑ in peak levels
MAOIs	Although not directly evaluated, serotonin syndrome (see GLOSSARY) possible when nefazodone used within 14 days of stopping MAOI therapy. Allow 7 days between stopping nefazodone and starting MAOI
Nonsedating antihistamines (astemizole)	Concurrent use absolutely contraindicated; ↑ risk of fatal ventricular arrhythmias

Abbreviations defined in GLOSSARY.

Information in this table obtained from *Physicians' Desk Reference, Facts and Comparisons,* or *AHFS Drug Information.* Please refer to those sources for current and additional prescribing information.

Nefazodone is rated Pregnancy Category C (see GLOSSARY; see also DRUG USE IN PREGNANCY/LACTATION, page 162); data on excretion in breast milk are lacking. Symptoms noted in overdose situations include nausea, vomiting, and somnolence; overdoses are not usually fatal.

Warnings/Precautions

Nefazodone is contraindicated for use with nonsedating antihistamines (eg, astemizole) and cisapride (see Table 57). Orthostatic hypotension and bradycardia can occur; use nefazodone carefully in patients with underlying cardiovascular disease or conditions that would predispose to hypotension. Like virtually all antidepressants, nefazodone may precipitate mania or hypomania in depressed patients.

Dosing Guidelines

Usual starting dose: Although 100 mg BID is recommended by the manufacturer, we recommend 50 mg BID and, in the elderly, 50 mg QD; increase by 50 to 100 mg/d after 1 week if tolerated. Maintain BID dosing schedule because of the short $t_{1/2}$. Dosage reductions are not needed for patients with renal impairment.

TRAZODONE

Table 58. Overview of trazodone therapy

Feature	Comments
Mechanism	5-HT$_2$-receptor antagonist; weak inhibitor of 5-HT, but not NE or DA reuptake. Active metabolite (m-CPP) is a direct postsynaptic 5-HT agonist. Little affinity for cholinergic receptors; strong α_1- but weak α_2-receptor antagonist[241]
Pharmacokinetics	Well absorbed, faster peak levels (1 h) in fasting state (but ↑ dizziness); BID dosing (t$_{1/2}$ 3 - 9 h). Extensively metabolized to major metabolite (m-CPP) that is eliminated more slowly and achieves higher plasma levels than parent compound. Clinical utility of plasma level monitoring not established. Little known about drug interactions
Efficacy	Major depression; useful in agitated/anxious depression and perhaps as anxiolytic in nondepressed patients who cannot use benzodiazepines. May be combined with SSRIs to treat persistent insomnia. Use in elderly limited by significant orthostatic hypotension
Safety	Significant sedation, orthostatic hypotension, dizziness, headache, nausea. Free of anticholinergic side effects. Serious: priapism (rare)
Dosing	50 or 100 mg HS; ↑ by 50 mg every 3 - 4 days to 200 - 400 mg/d (BID schedule). Maximum in severe depression 600 mg/d (BID or TID). Anxiolytic activity may occur within 1 - 2 weeks

Abbreviations defined in GLOSSARY.

Efficacy

Trazodone (Desyrel®) is an effective antidepressant.[247,248] Because it causes significant sedation, it may be most useful in agitated or anxious depressed patients or perhaps in anxious nondepressed patients in whom benzodiazepines cannot be used.[249] The use of trazodone for geriatric depression may be limited by significant orthostatic hypotension.[241] Trazodone also has been studied in PD, agoraphobia, and BN[250] but efficacy data are not compelling.

Drug Interactions

Few drug interactions have been reported (Table 59).

Table 59. Common drug interactions with trazodone

Interacting drug	Effect of interaction
Alcohol, CNS depressants	↑ Drowsiness, sedation
Clonidine	↓ Antihypertensive effect; avoid concurrent use. Also may need ↓ dose of other antihypertensive agents because of orthostatic hypotension caused by trazodone
MAOIs	Serotonin syndrome (see GLOSSARY) possible when trazodone used within 14 days of stopping MAOI therapy. May be dose related (seen at doses ≥150 mg/d), but combination generally not recommended. Allow 7 days between stopping trazodone and starting MAOI

Abbreviations defined in GLOSSARY.

Information in this table obtained from *Physicians' Desk Reference, Facts and Comparisons,* or *AHFS Drug Information.* Please refer to those sources for current and additional prescribing information.

Safety

Significant sedation is common and can be a treatment-limiting side effect. However, this feature may be advantageous in anxious or agitated depressed patients, in those with insomnia, or in those with SSRI-induced activation. Orthostatic hypotension, dizziness, headache, and nausea are common. Trazodone is relatively free of the anticholinergic side effects common to TCAs. Priapism occurs rarely (1 in 5000 to 1 in 6000), but trazodone is the most common priapism-inducing drug. This condition may require surgical intervention or cause permanent loss of erectile function. The risk is highest in the first month of treatment; discontinue trazodone immediately if abnormal erectile function occurs.

In overdose situations, significant hypotension is a prominent symptom, but even with very large doses (9.2 g), fatalities are infrequent unless other drugs are ingested simultaneously.[241] Trazodone is rated Pregnancy Category C (see GLOSSARY; see also DRUG USE IN PREGNANCY/LACTATION, page 162) and probably is excreted in breast milk.

Warnings/Precautions

Case reports suggest trazodone may be arrhythmogenic in the early post-MI phase; monitor patients with underlying cardiac disease while they are on trazodone.[241]

Dosing Guidelines

Usual starting dose: 50 or 100 mg HS; increase by 50 mg every 3 to 4 days to 200 to 400 mg/d (divided BID). More severely depressed patients may require up to 600 mg/d (divided BID or TID) although this dose is often not well tolerated. Clinical benefit (anxiolytic activity) may occur within 1 to 2 weeks.

VENLAFAXINE

Table 60. Overview of venlafaxine therapy

Feature	Comments
Mechanism	Blocks 5-HT and NE reuptake (5-HT > NE), weakly blocks DA reuptake. Major metabolite inhibits NE and 5-HT reuptake. Lacks activity at histamine, cholinergic, or α- or β-adrenergic receptors[244,251]
Pharmacokinetics	Peak levels within 2 h (immediate-release formulation), within 6 h (extended-release formulation). Effects of food are variable[251]; ≤30% protein bound. Highly metabolized via CYP2D6; one major, two minor active metabolites. Immediate-release formulation dosed BID/TID ($t_{1/2}$ <10 h), extended-release formulation dosed QD. ↓ Clearance in severe renal or hepatic impairment. No therapeutic plasma range; few drug interactions reported but ↑ haloperidol levels
Efficacy	Short-term: similar to TCAs, trazodone, fluoxetine. Limited comparative data with other antidepressants. May be particularly effective in severe depression. Effective in GAD. Other psychiatric indications being studied
Safety	Nausea, vomiting, headache, dizziness, anxiety, anorexia, insomnia, sweating. Sexual dysfunction, weight loss occur. Dose-related ↑ BP (10 - 15 mm Hg), heart rate. Abrupt cessation results in discontinuation syndrome. ↑ QT_c with extended-release formulation
Dosing	75 mg/d with food divided BID or TID; ↑ by ≤75 mg/d not more often than every 4 days after response is assessed (maximum 375 mg/d). New extended-release form may be dosed QD (morning) at same dose level. Monitor BP regularly. ↓ Dose by 50% in hepatic impairment and by 25% in renal impairment

Abbreviations defined in GLOSSARY.

Efficacy

Short-term antidepressant efficacy of venlafaxine (Effexor®) is comparable to some TCAs, trazodone, and fluoxetine.[251-253] Large-scale postmarketing comparative clinical experience with SSRIs is currently under study. Like other antidepressants, the onset of clinical activity is often delayed for 2 weeks or longer.[251] Venlafaxine has not been widely studied for other psychiatric indications except for generalized anxiety disorder (GAD). The extended-release formulation (Effexor®XR) also is effective for major depression.[254]

Drug Interactions

Venlafaxine is both metabolized by and inhibits the CYP2D6 isoenzyme, but it appears to be a much weaker inhibitor than SSRIs.[213] Limited data suggest no interactions with lithium, alcohol, or diazepam.[251] Like other agents that inhibit serotonin reuptake, however, venlafaxine should not be used concurrently with MAOIs.

Safety

Venlafaxine is relatively well tolerated, especially the new extended-release form. As with SSRIs, nausea, vomiting, headache, dizziness, anxiety, anorexia, insomnia, and sweating are common side effects of venlafaxine. Nausea and dizziness dissipate with continued therapy. Sexual dysfunction may be dose related, but it occurs somewhat less often than with SSRIs.[241] Weight loss may be significant. The incidence of anticholinergic, CNS, and cardiac conduction side effects is very much lower with venlafaxine than with TCAs. The extended-release form of venlafaxine has been reported to increase QT_c intervals; this has not been reported with the immediate-release product. Venlafaxine causes modest dose-related elevations in BP (10 to 15 mm Hg increase in supine diastolic BP) and heart rate (4 bpm) that are probably not clinically significant in otherwise healthy depressed patients but that may be clinically relevant in hypertensive patients.[252] The effect is dose related, with 13% of patients taking 300 mg/d or more demonstrating significant elevations in blood pressure. Venlafaxine overdoses are typically nonfatal; somnolence was the most common symptom reported. Venlafaxine is rated Pregnancy Category C (see GLOSSARY; see also DRUG USE IN PREGNANCY/ LACTATION, page 162); data on excretion in breast milk are not yet available.

Warnings/Precautions

Venlafaxine is contraindicated for use with MAOIs; allow at least 14 days between stopping MAOI therapy and initiating venlafaxine. Use cautiously in patients with seizure disorders or a history of the same.

Dosing Guidelines

Usual starting dose of immediate-release form: 75 mg/d (divided BID or TID) taken with food. Increase by 75 mg/d or less to a dose of 150 mg/d and then to 225 mg/d not more often than every 4 days after response is assessed. For severely depressed patients, the maximum dose is 375 mg/d. Routine BP monitoring is suggested for all patients. Reduce the dose by 50% in patients with moderate hepatic impairment and by about 25% in those with moderate renal impairment. Dosage reductions are not needed in otherwise healthy elderly depressed patients. The extended-release form can be administered once daily, preferably in the morning. Dosing targets are a recommended maximum of 225 mg/d, but some patients require the same doses as with the immediate-release form. Withdrawal of venlafaxine, either as immediate- or extended-release formulations, should be gradual.

Drugs for Bipolar Disorder

Three mood-stabilizing drugs, lithium carbonate, carbamazepine, and valproic acid, are used to manage acute mania and also play an important role in the treatment of bipolar depression and in the long-term management of bipolar disorder.

LITHIUM

For nearly 50 years, lithium has been known to be useful for the treatment of mania (Table 61).

Table 61. Overview of lithium therapy

Feature	Comments
Mechanism	Complex and not fully understood; alters sodium ion transport, ↑ NE reuptake and 5-HT transmission, second-messenger systems, gene expression. Also may correct desynchronized circadian rhythms[255]
Pharmacokinetics	Good oral absorption, unaffected by food. Peak levels in 1 - 4 h; long $t_{1/2}$ (24 h). Crosses blood-brain barrier, not protein bound, not metabolized, renally excreted. Therapeutic range 0.8 - 1.2 mEq/L. Drug interactions common
Efficacy	Acute mania, prophylaxis of bipolar disorder. Also acute bipolar depression and augmentation in resistant depression
Safety	Narrow therapeutic index. Therapeutic range: 0.8 - 1.2 mEq/L. Fine hand tremor, polyuria, mild excessive thirst, drowsiness, ↑ weight, transient nausea, memory problems, diarrhea
Dosing	Initial dose: 300 mg TID, ↑ by 300 mg/d every few days until response or therapeutic level. Lower initial doses in elderly or patients with renal dysfunction. Usual range: 600 mg TID (900 mg BID sustained-release). Monitor serum levels twice weekly until stable, then weekly to avoid toxicity and maximize efficacy. In maintenance (300 mg TID or QID), monitor levels every 2 or 3 months (more often in elderly). Regularly monitor renal status, TFTs, electrolytes, hematologic status, glucose, ECG

Abbreviations defined in GLOSSARY.

Efficacy

Lithium is used in acute mania, but because clinical response is delayed about 1 to 2 weeks, benzodiazepines, antipsychotics, or certain anticonvulsants are helpful in the early stages of a manic episode. Up to 80% of patients show at least some response to lithium. Lithium also is used as prophylaxis against subsequent manic episodes in recurrent bipolar illness; it reduces the frequency and severity of the episodes.[255,256] Lithium may be useful for acute treatment of bipolar depression and has been used as an augmentation strategy for resistant depression.[255,257] Lithium may be less effective for dysphoric mania (mixed state) or rapid cycling disorder.

Drug Interactions

Lithium is involved with a number of serious drug interactions (Table 62).

Table 62. Common drug interactions with lithium[255]

Interacting drug	Effect of interaction
Antiarrhythmics	May alter cardiac conduction
Antipsychotics	May ↑ lithium toxicity even with normal lithium levels. Rare encephalopathic syndrome (weakness, lethargy, fever, ↑ EPS, confusion) with irreversible brain damage may be same as NMS; may be more common with high-potency antipsychotics (eg, haloperidol)
Bupropion	May ↑ seizure risk
Carbamazepine	↑ Neurotoxic effects with normal lithium levels
Thiazide diuretics	↓ Lithium clearance: ↑ lithium levels; loop or potassium-sparing diuretics may be safer
Iodide salts	May ↑ risk of hypothyroidism
Methyldopa	↑ Toxicity with high or normal lithium levels
Metronidazole	May ↑ lithium levels
Neuromuscular blockers	Severe respiratory depression possible
NSAIDs	↓ Lithium renal clearance: ↑ lithium levels; monitor lithium levels
SSRIs	Lithium may ↑ serotonergic effects of SSRIs
Sympathomimetic amines[a]	↓ Pressor sensitivity possible
TCAs	↑ Pharmacologic effects of TCAs
Theophylline	↑ Lithium renal excretion: ↓ lithium levels; monitor levels
Urinary alkalinizers	↑ Lithium renal clearance: ↓ lithium levels
Verapamil	↑ Or ↓ lithium levels; monitor levels

Abbreviations defined in GLOSSARY.

[a]Dextromethorphan, ephedrine, levarterenol, mephentermine, methylphenidate, phenylephrine, phenylpropanolamine, pseudoephedrine.

Information in this table obtained from *Physicians' Desk Reference, Facts and Comparisons*, or *AHFS Drug Information*. Please refer to those sources for current and additional prescribing information.

Safety

The side-effect profile of lithium affects nearly every organ system.[255] Because lithium and sodium compete for reabsorption in the kidneys, in sodium-depleted states (eg, diuretic use, dehydration), lithium is resorbed and serum levels rise, possibly leading to toxicity. Conversely, sodium loading causes serum lithium levels to fall.

Common adverse events include fine hand tremor, polyuria, mild excessive thirst, drowsiness, weight gain, transient nausea, diarrhea, and memory problems. Most occur during titration but some may persist. Lithium has a very narrow therapeutic index; toxic or disabling effects are infrequent with serum levels of 1.5 mEq/L or lower although some elderly patients demonstrate significant side effects at these levels. Mild or moderate adverse events occur with serum levels between 1.5 and 2.5 mEq/L, and moderate to severe side effects occur with levels of 2.0 to 2.5 mEq/L. Acute withdrawal of lithium may precipitate a manic episode. Side effects unrelated to serum levels include ECG changes (flat T waves), bradycardia, edema, transient hyperglycemia, pruritus with or without rash, leukocytosis, and headache. Lithium is rated Pregnancy Category D (see GLOSSARY; see also DRUG USE IN PREGNANCY/LACTATION, page 162) and may cause significant toxicity in newborns; do not use in nursing mothers.

Warnings/Precautions

Lithium toxicity is high, and serum levels must be monitored very frequently in patients with underlying renal or cardiac disease (or in those taking drugs that may cause bradycardia [eg, ß-blockers]), in severely debilitated patients, and in patients in states of dehydration, sodium depletion, or diuretic use. Because of normal reductions in renal function associated with aging, the elderly are particularly sensitive to toxic effects of lithium. Patients must avoid dehydration through adequate fluid (2.5 to 3 L/d) and dietary sodium intake. Chronic lithium treatment may cause interstitial renal changes, acquired nephrogenic diabetes insipidus, or hypothyroidism (with long-term use).

Dosing and Monitoring Guidelines

A regimen of 600 mg TID or 900 mg BID (sustained-release) usually provides serum lithium levels of 1.0 to 1.5 mEq/L. Initiate therapy with 300 mg TID and increase by 300 mg/d every 4 to 5 days until response or therapeutic level. In the elderly, start at 300 mg/d and aim for doses between 900 and 1200 mg/d. The onset of therapeutic effect is in 1 to 2 weeks. Monitor serum levels 12 hours after the evening dose at least twice weekly during stabilization and weekly thereafter. The desirable serum-level range for maintenance therapy is 0.8 to 1.2 mEq/L; a dose of 300 mg TID or QID will usually provide this range. During maintenance, check levels every 2 or 3 months (more frequently for elderly patients). Regularly (at least every 6 months) monitor renal function (eg, creatinine clearance [CrCl]), electrolytes, thyroid function, hematologic status, fasting glucose, and ECG status.

CARBAMAZEPINE

The antiepileptic agent carbamazepine (Tegretol®) (Table 63) may be used in bipolar illness if lithium or valproate is ineffective or poorly tolerated, or in patients in whom these FDA-approved drugs may not be appropriate (eg, severe renal impairment). It is structurally related to TCAs.

Table 63. Overview of carbamazepine therapy

Feature	Comments
Mechanism	Mechanism in mania unknown; unclear if antiepileptic and mood-stabilizing actions are related.[258] Binds and inactivates sodium ion channels to ↓ rapid high-frequency action potential firing. Also blocks NE uptake, but does not block DA receptors; binds to peripheral benzodiazepine receptors
Pharmacokinetics	Erratic oral absorption (anticholinergic properties may ↓ GI transit time), peak in 4 - 8 h but may be delayed for >24 h, ≤85% protein bound. Highly metabolized via CYP450; one active metabolite (causes neurotoxicity). $t_{1/2}$ 18 - 55 h; may induce its own metabolism with chronic treatment. Clinically significant drug interactions
Efficacy	Acute mania in lithium-intolerant or -resistant patients
Safety	Dose-related, transient diplopia, blurry vision, fatigue, vertigo, nausea, vomiting, ataxia. Also, hyponatremia, skin rash, transient leukopenia, thrombocytopenia, ↑ LFTs. Rare idiosyncratic agranulocytosis, aplastic anemia, hepatic failure, Stevens-Johnson syndrome
Dosing	100 mg QD or BID with meals to ↓ GI upset; ↑ by 100 - 200 mg every few days as tolerated (to 2 g/d) to achieve serum levels of 6 - 10 µg/mL

Abbreviations defined in GLOSSARY.

Efficacy

Carbamazepine is not approved by the FDA for acute mania, but it may be effective for this use in lithium-intolerant or -resistant patients. Response rates in acute mania are similar to lithium and antipsychotics; onset of clinical effect may be faster with carbamazepine than with lithium. Factors predicting good response to carbamazepine include severe mania, rapid cycling (≥4 episodes/y), and greater dysphoria or depression during mania.[258] Carbamazepine also has been studied for treatment of acute unipolar or bipolar depression.[258]

Drug Interactions

Carbamazepine causes several clinically important drug interactions related to induction or inhibition of hepatic-metabolizing enzymes (CYP3A4 and probably others) (Table 64).

Table 64. Common drug interactions with carbamazepine[258]

Interacting drug	Effect of interaction
Anticoagulants	↑ Warfarin metabolism: ↓ efficacy
Antipsychotics	↓ Haloperidol levels: ↓ efficacy; also ↑ neurotoxicity; ↑ risk of leukopenia (clozapine)
Barbiturates	↓ Carbamazepine levels: ↓ efficacy
Benzodiazepines	Carbamazepine ↑ metabolism and ↓ levels of alprazolam, clonazepam
Bupropion	Carbamazepine may ↓ bupropion levels
Calcium channel blockers	Diltiazem, verapamil ↓ carbamazepine metabolism: ↑ levels, toxicity
Lithium	↑ Neurotoxicity
Macrolide antimicrobials	Erythromycin, others (not azithromycin) ↓ carbamazepine metabolism: ↑ levels, toxicity
MAOIs	Concurrent use contraindicated; allow ≥14 days between discontinuation of MAOI and initiation of carbamazepine
Nefazodone	↑ Carbamazepine levels: ↑ toxicity
Oral contraceptives	↓ Contraceptive efficacy
Phenytoin	↓ Carbamazepine levels; ↑ or ↓ phenytoin levels; monitor levels
SSRIs	Fluoxetine, fluvoxamine may ↑ carbamazepine levels: ↑ toxicity
TCAs	↑ Carbamazepine levels: ↑ toxicity; ↓ TCA levels
Theophylline	↓ Carbamazepine levels and ↑ or ↓ theophylline levels; monitor levels
Valproic acid	↓ Valproic acid levels, ↑ carbamazepine levels

Abbreviations defined in GLOSSARY.

Information in this table obtained from *Physicians' Desk Reference, Facts and Comparisons*, or *AHFS Drug Information*. Please refer to those sources for current and additional prescribing information.

Safety

Carbamazepine causes fewer renal side effects and perhaps less memory impairment than lithium, although its side-effect profile is far from optimal. Common, dose-related, and transient side effects include diplopia, blurry vision, fatigue, vertigo, nausea, vomiting, and ataxia. Use of low initial doses may minimize these early side effects. In overdose, neuromuscular (coma, convulsions) symptoms are most prominent and cardiac symptoms occur only with very high doses (>60 g).

Carbamazepine is rated Pregnancy Category C (see GLOSSARY; see also DRUG USE IN PREGNANCY/LACTATION, page 162); teratogenic effects occur but prophylactic folic acid prior to conception may reduce the frequency of some birth defects (eg, neural tube defects). The drug passes into breast milk and accumulates in fetal tissue; assess whether discontinuation of the drug or of nursing is more beneficial to the mother.

Warnings/Precautions

Carbamazepine is contraindicated in patients with previous bone marrow depression. Carbamazepine causes a transient leukopenia and thrombocytopenia (unrelated to aplastic anemia or agranulocytosis) in up to 12% of patients. Rarely, however, it causes idiosyncratic agranulocytosis or aplastic anemia in the first 6 months of therapy. Elevated LFTs occur in up to 15% of patients; hepatic failure occurs rarely. Cardiac conduction disturbances also may occur rarely. These side effects are managed by dose reductions or discontinuation of therapy and the drug can be restarted once hematologic and hepatic indices normalize. Periodically monitor LFTs, urine, and blood urea nitrogen (BUN); baseline hematologic indices (ie, complete blood count [CBC] with differential, platelets) with monthly checks for the first 2 months of therapy are needed. Thereafter, check every 6 months to yearly.

Steroid-responsive skin rash does not require discontinuation of therapy if there is no bleeding or exfoliation (ie, Stevens-Johnson syndrome). Carbamazepine may increase antidiuretic hormone and cause hyponatremia in up to 30% of patients; the elderly are more prone to developing this effect and often must be withdrawn from therapy. Mild anticholinergic activity may worsen angle-closure glaucoma.

Dosing Guidelines

Usual starting dose: 100 mg QD or BID; increase every few days by 100 to 200 mg as tolerated (up to 2 g/d) to achieve serum levels between 6 and 10 µg/mL. Take with meals to reduce GI upset.

VALPROIC ACID

The antiepileptic valproic acid is an alternative to carbamazepine for lithium-intolerant or -resistant patients with mania or bipolar illness (Table 65). In contrast to carbamazepine, valproate is FDA-approved for the acute treatment of mania. Four oral products are available: valproic acid capsules and sodium valproate oral syrup (both known as Depakene®) and enteric-coated, sustained-release divalproex sodium tablets and oral sprinkle capsules (both known as Depakote®); divalproex is the most commonly used form of valproic acid. Doses are reported as valproic acid because this is what is found in plasma.

Table 65. Overview of valproic acid therapy

Feature	Comments
Mechanism	Unknown; may ↓ GABA catabolism, ↑ GABA release, ↓ GABA turnover, or ↑ GABA-receptor density. Also affects sodium ion transport, does not bind to benzodiazepine receptors. May ↓ DA turnover
Pharmacokinetics	Peak level in 2 h (immediate-release) and 3 - 8 h (sustained-release); food may ↓ absorption. Highly protein bound, highly metabolized via oxidation and CYP450 to active and inactive metabolites. $t_{1/2}$ 5 - 20 h. Effective serum levels 50 - 150 µg/mL. Significant drug interactions
Efficacy	Acute mania (similar to lithium); ↑ efficacy in rapid cycling (≥4 episodes/y) and ↑ dysphoria or depression during mania. Used for prophylaxis of bipolar disorder
Safety	Nausea, somnolence, dizziness, vomiting, weakness, dyspepsia, skin rash. Serious: hepatic failure, thrombocytopenia, abnormal coagulation parameters
Dosing	Divalproex sustained-release: 750 mg/d (divided); ↑ as tolerated to desired effect or to serum level of 50 - 150 µg/mL. Maximum 60 mg/kg/d. Take with food or H_2-receptor antagonist to ↓ GI upset. Do not chew tablets. ↓ Dose in elderly

Abbreviations defined in GLOSSARY.

Efficacy

Valproic acid is as effective as lithium for the treatment of acute mania;[259] divalproex sodium sustained-release tablets are FDA-indicated for this use. Factors predicting good response to valproic acid include rapid cycling (≥4 episodes/y), greater dysphoria or depression during mania, later age at onset, and shorter duration of the condition.[258] The threshold plasma level for clinical benefit appears to be 50 µg/mL; some manic patients may require levels higher than 100 mg/mL, whereas hypomanic patients may respond at levels less than 50 µg/mL.[258] Valproic acid may be effective for prophylaxis of bipolar disorder or for acute bipolar depression. In addition to bipolar disorder, valproic acid also is used to treat a variety of symptoms that cut across diagnostic entities. These include the aggression, impulsivity, and agitation associated with a broad range of disorders including Alzheimer's disease and other dementias, intermittent compulsive disorders, childhood disorders (eg, autism), and others.

Drug Interactions

Common drug interactions with valproic acid are shown below (Table 66). Valproic acid may interfere with urine ketone tests; TFTs also may be altered.

Table 66. Common drug interactions with valproic acid[258]

Interacting drug	Effect of interaction
Anticoagulants	May ↑ unbound (free) warfarin: ↑ hypoprothrombinemic effects; monitor PT
Aspirin (chronic or high-dose)	May displace valproic acid from protein-binding sites: ↑ levels, toxicity
Bupropion	May ↑ valproic acid levels
Carbamazepine	↑ Carbamazepine levels, ↓ valproic acid levels
Chlorpromazine	↑ Valproic acid $t_{1/2}$, ↑ trough levels, ↓ clearance
Cimetidine	↑ Valproic acid $t_{1/2}$, ↓ clearance
Diazepam	↓ Diazepam metabolism, ↑ CNS effects
Erythromycin	↑ Valproic acid levels: ↑ toxicity
Fluoxetine	↑ Valproic acid levels
Lamotrigine	↓ Valproic acid levels, ↑ lamotrigine levels; may need to ↓ lamotrigine dose
Phenobarbital	↓ Phenobarbital metabolism: ↑ levels; ↑ valproic acid clearance: ↓ levels
Phenytoin	↑ Action of phenytoin even with therapeutic levels. ↑ Valproic acid metabolism: ↓ efficacy
TCAs	↑ TCA levels possible
Tolbutamide	↑ Unbound (free) tolbutamide, significance unknown
Zidovudine	↓ Zidovudine clearance in HIV+ patients

Abbreviations defined in GLOSSARY.

Information in this table obtained from *Physicians' Desk Reference, Facts and Comparisons,* or *AHFS Drug Information.* Please refer to those sources for current and additional prescribing information.

Safety

Common side effects include nausea, somnolence, dizziness, vomiting, weakness, dyspepsia, tremor, and skin rash. Transient hair loss, weight gain, and increased appetite (and associated weight gain) may occur. Overall, valproic acid is better tolerated by manic patients than is lithium. Valproic acid is rated Pregnancy Category D (see GLOSSARY; see also DRUG USE IN PREGNANCY/LACTATION, page 162); its use during pregnancy is associated with an increased rate of neural tube defects (spina bifida). Use of folic acid (4 mg) during pregnancy is useful if this therapy is to be continued. Valproic acid passes into breast milk but effects on the infant are not known; use cautiously in nursing mothers. In overdose, valproic acid causes heart block, coma, and somnolence; fatalities have occurred.

Warnings/Precautions

Valproic acid is contraindicated in hepatic disease or dysfunction. The drug can cause fatal hepatic failure; the risk is dose related, is greatest in younger children (especially those taking other antiepileptics), and decreases with age. Hepatic failure has not been reported in adults on valproic acid monotherapy. Monitor patients for malaise, weakness, facial edema, and jaundice, and check LFTs at baseline and frequently during the first 6 months of therapy. Note that LFTs may be normal, however. Valproic acid also can cause thrombocytopenia and abnormal coagulation parameters; check these at baseline and periodically during treatment, although they too may be normal and do not predict hematologic problems.

Dosing Guidelines

Usual starting dose (divalproex sodium enteric-coated, sustained-release tablets): 500 to 750 mg/d in divided doses; increase as rapidly as tolerated to desired effect (serum level 50 to 150 µg/mL). In acute mania, a more rapid response may be obtained by giving 20 to 30 mg/kg, thus reducing the need for antipsychotic or benzodiazepine use.[258] The elderly may require lower doses. Maximum: 60 mg/kg/d. Advise patient to take with food or H_2-receptor antagonist (not cimetidine), if needed, to reduce GI upset, and not to chew tablets.

Benzodiazepines

All benzodiazepines have anxiolytic, hypnotic, muscle-relaxant, and anti-convulsant properties. Superficial designations (indications) such as an *anxiolytic* or *hypnotic* benzodiazepine are for marketing purposes only. Only oral products used to manage anxiety disorders and insomnia are reviewed herein (Table 67); injectable products primarily used for acute alcohol withdrawal, seizures, tetanus, or anesthesia (ie, chlordiazepoxide, diazepam, midazolam, lorazepam) are not considered.

Table 67. Overview of oral benzodiazepine therapy

Feature	Comments
Mechanism	Facilitate GABA transmission via nonselective binding to benzodiazepine receptors adjacent to $GABA_A$ receptor sites within the GABA complex. BZ_1 receptor associated with sleep; BZ_2 with motor function, memory, cognition
Pharmacokinetics	Good oral absorption; peak levels in 0.5 - 6 h. 70% to >90% protein bound, lipid soluble (readily cross blood-brain and placental barriers). Extensive metabolism (Table 68), many with active metabolites (agents with inactive metabolites preferred in elderly or patients with liver impairment); drug interactions common
Efficacy	Effective anxiolytics and hypnotics; base selection on pharmacokinetic features or cost
Safety	Wide safety margin in therapeutic or overdose situations. Transient, dose-related drowsiness. Memory impairment or confusion in elderly. Even short-term use (≤6 weeks) may cause physical dependence or withdrawal syndrome upon abrupt discontinuation
Dosing	Individualize; ↑ gradually. Use low initial doses and ↑ gradually to ↓ risk of hypotension in elderly

Abbreviations defined in GLOSSARY.

Table 68. Comparative features of oral benzodiazepines[260,261]

Drug	Dose range (mg/d)	Tmax (h)	$t_{1/2}$[a]	Major metabolic pathway	Clinically active metabolite?
Alprazolam (Xanax®)	0.75 - 4[b]	1 - 2	I	Oxidation	No
Chlordiazepoxide (Librium®)	15 - 100	0.5 - 4	L	Oxidation	Yes
Clonazepam (Klonopin®)	1.5 - 20	1 - 2	L	Oxidation	No
Clorazepate (Tranxene®)	15 - 60	1 - 2	L	Oxidation	Yes
Diazepam (Valium®)	4 - 40	0.5 - 2	L	Oxidation	Yes
Estazolam (ProSom™)	1 - 2	2	I	Oxidation	No
Flurazepam (Dalmane®)	15 - 30	0.5 - 1	L	Oxidation	Yes
Lorazepam (Ativan®)	2 - 4	1 - 6	I	Glucuronidation	No
Oxazepam (Serax®)	30 - 120	2 - 6	I	Glucuronidation	No
Quazepam (Doral®)	15	2	L	Oxidation	Yes
Temazepam (Restoril®)	15 - 30	2 - 4	I	Glucuronidation	No
Triazolam (Halcion®)	0.125 - 0.5	0.5 - 2	S	Oxidation	No

Abbreviations defined in GLOSSARY.

[a] I = intermediate (6 - 20 h); L = long (>20 h); S = short (<6 h); parent and active metabolites (if present).

[b] Higher doses (1.5 - 10 mg/d) may be needed for PD.

Information in this table obtained from *Physicians' Desk Reference*, *Facts and Comparisons*, or *AHFS Drug Information*. Please refer to those sources for current and additional prescribing information.

Psychopharmacologic Agents

Efficacy

All benzodiazepines are similarly and highly effective for relief of anxiety and insomnia;[261] base drug selection on pharmacokinetic features or cost (most are available as generic products). Benzodiazepines decrease sleep latency (ie, the time to get to sleep), time spent awake (Stage 0 sleep), number of awakenings, and REM sleep; the net result is an increase in total sleep time. For short-term management of insomnia, benzodiazepines are effective, but use is limited to a few weeks. For anxiety disorders, periodically assess the need for drug therapy after about 4 or 6 months. Benzodiazepines are not routinely effective for the treatment of depression and, in some cases, may precipitate or exacerbate depressive symptoms.

Drug Interactions

Most drug interactions with benzodiazepines are related to their extensive hepatic metabolism (Table 69). Drugs that inhibit hepatic metabolism (eg, cimetidine, oral contraceptives, disulfiram, fluvoxamine, isoniazid, ketoconazole, metoprolol, nefazodone, propranolol, propoxyphene, and valproic acid) reduce the elimination of benzodiazepines that are metabolized through oxidative pathways (see Table 68) and increase pharmacologic effects (ie, sedation, impaired psychomotor functioning). Reported laboratory test interferences include false-negative urine glucose tests (Clinistix, Diastix), false-positive pregnancy tests, and interference with urinary steroid analyses.

Safety

Benzodiazepines have a wide safety margin with little effect on cardiovascular and respiratory systems in therapeutic doses as well as overdoses (when ingested without alcohol or other drugs). Common, predictable side effects (eg, sedation, dizziness) are an extension of their pharmacologic properties and may be exacerbated when benzodiazepines are taken with alcohol. Drowsiness is usually mild and transient. To reduce the risk of falls in the elderly, increase doses gradually and reduce the dose if drowsiness, confusion, and ataxia are pronounced. Other less common side effects include nausea, constipation or diarrhea, changes in libido, bradycardia or tachycardia, visual disturbances, pruritus, hiccoughs, fever, and diaphoresis. Rebound insomnia (ie, insomnia that is worse than pretreatment insomnia) upon discontinuation of therapy can occur.[262] See specific prescribing information for full safety information.

During long-term therapy, perform periodic blood counts and LFTs to detect jaundice and neutropenia. Anxiolytic benzodiazepines are rated Pregnancy Category D; flurazepam and triazolam are Category X (see GLOSSARY; see also DRUG USE IN PREGNANCY/LACTATION, page 162). Benzodiazepines cross the placenta and accumulate in fetal circulation; an increased risk of congenital malformations (cleft palate) has been observed when these drugs (specifically, diazepam) were used in the first trimester. Because they pass into breast milk, do not give benzodiazepines to nursing mothers.

Table 69. Common drug interactions with benzodiazepines

Interacting drug	Effect of interaction
Alcohol, CNS depressants	↑ CNS depression
Antacids	May alter rate but not extent of absorption; stagger administration times
Fluvoxamine, nefazodone	Inhibit metabolism of alprazolam, triazolam; may ↑ levels, ↑ elimination $t_{1/2}$, ↑ CNS depression
Oral contraceptives	May ↑ clearance of glucuronidated benzodiazepines; may ↓ metabolism of oxidized benzodiazepines
Digoxin	↑ Digoxin serum levels; monitor serum levels
Levodopa	Benzodiazepines may ↓ efficacy of levodopa
Macrolide antimicrobials	↑ Triazolam bioavailability, ↓ triazolam clearance
Phenytoin, carbamazepine	Anticonvulsant levels may ↑; monitor
Probenecid	May interfere with benzodiazepine metabolism; faster onset of action or prolonged effects
Ranitidine	↓ GI absorption of diazepam
Rifampin	↑ Benzodiazepine metabolism: ↓ therapeutic effects
Theophylline	May antagonize sedative effects of benzodiazepines

Abbreviations defined in GLOSSARY.

Information in this table obtained from *Physicians' Desk Reference, Facts and Comparisons,* or *AHFS Drug Information.* Please refer to those sources for current and additional prescribing information.

Warnings/Precautions

Benzodiazepine use for as little as 4 to 6 weeks can lead to physical dependence and a withdrawal syndrome upon discontinuation.[261] This syndrome is more likely with short-acting agents, with regular use for 3 months or more, and when discontinuation is abrupt. Typical withdrawal symptoms include anxiety, flu-like illness, restlessness, sweating, insomnia, irritability, muscle tension/cramps, and anorexia. More major symptoms include confusion, depersonalization, hallucinations, abnormal perception of movement, and psychosis. Grand mal seizures and status epilepticus have occurred in patients withdrawing from alprazolam or clonazepam therapy. Gradual dose reduction over 1 to 2 months is recommended. Patients on short-acting agents can be switched to longer-acting agents during this time to facilitate discontinuation.

In depressed patients with suicidal tendencies who also are anxious, prescribe and dispense only small amounts of drug. Although fatal overdoses have not been documented with benzodiazepines alone, they have occurred when these drugs were part of a multidrug ingestion, usually with alcohol. Some benzodiazepines (clonazepam, diazepam, clorazepate) may paradoxically increase seizure frequency in patients with underlying seizure disorders; patients taking these products should carry medical identification.

Dosing Guidelines

Individualize initial dosing and increase doses gradually. For anxiety disorders, multiple daily doses are usually needed; however, single HS doses of clorazepate or clonazepam can be used. In the elderly, use low initial doses and increase gradually to minimize any risk of hypotension. Single daily doses may be appropriate for some elderly patients.

Nonbenzodiazepine Anxiolytics

This miscellaneous group of anti-anxiety agents includes buspirone (BuSpar®) (Table 70) and meprobamate (Miltown®, Equanil®).

BUSPIRONE

Table 70. Overview of buspirone therapy

Feature	Comments
Mechanism	Partial agonist at 5-HT$_{1A}$ receptors, some affinity for D$_2$ receptors, may ↑ NE metabolism. No clinical effects on benzodiazepine-GABA receptors
Pharmacokinetics	Rapid oral absorption (peak levels within 40 - 90 min), 95% protein bound. Extensively metabolized; one active metabolite (1-PP). BID dosing (t$_{1/2}$ 2 - 3 h [range 1 - 10 h]). Drug interactions infrequent
Efficacy	Comparable to benzodiazepines for GAD but slower acting (not for acute relief); lacks sedative, muscle relaxant, or anticonvulsant actions. No effect on benzodiazepine withdrawal symptoms. May be effective in augmenting antidepressant action. May reverse SSRI-induced sexual dysfunction
Dosing	15 mg/d (7.5 mg BID) for 1 week; ↑ by 5 mg every few days as tolerated to 30 mg/d (divided). Maximum 60 mg/d. Improvement in 2 weeks; optimal benefit in 4 - 7 weeks

Abbreviations defined in GLOSSARY.

Efficacy

Buspirone is comparable to benzodiazepines for the management of GAD and perhaps other chronic anxiety states. Long-term efficacy (>1 y) is maintained without the need for dosage increases. Its slow onset of action (4 to 7 weeks) precludes its use for acute anxiety relief. Buspirone may be ineffective in anxious patients who previously have used benzodiazepines.[263] One reason may be that buspirone does not relieve benzodiazepine withdrawal symptoms, so patients transferring from benzodiazepine therapy to buspirone may experience a resurgence of anxiety-like symptoms. Buspirone may be added to benzodiazepine therapy for several weeks before tapering the latter.[263] At doses higher than those used for GAD, buspirone may have limited antidepressant activity.[264]

Drug Interactions

Few clinically important drug interactions have been reported with buspirone (Table 71). It does not potentiate the CNS depressant effects of alcohol and can be used concomitantly with SSRIs.

Table 71. Common drug interactions with buspirone[263,265]

Interacting drug	Effect of interaction
Cyclosporin-A	↑ Cyclosporin-A levels: nephrotoxicity; monitor cyclosporin-A levels
Erythromycin	↓ Buspirone metabolism: ↑ plasma levels
Haloperidol	↑ Haloperidol levels
Itraconazole	↓ Buspirone metabolism: ↑ plasma levels
MAOIs	Buspirone may ↑ BP; avoid concurrent use with MAOIs

Abbreviations defined in GLOSSARY.

Information in this table obtained from *Physicians' Desk Reference, Facts and Comparisons,* or *AHFS Drug Information.* Please refer to those sources for current and additional prescribing information.

Safety

Buspirone is well tolerated; tolerance usually develops to common dose-related side effects of dizziness, headache, nausea, nervousness, lightheadedness, and agitation. Sexual dysfunction is infrequent and this drug may be useful to treat SSRI-induced sexual dysfunction. Unlike benzodiazepines, buspirone does not impair psychomotor performance, it is nonsedating, and has no effect on respiration. Buspirone has little effect on prolactin, cortisol, or growth hormone secretion.[263] The drug lacks abuse potential; neither tolerance nor a withdrawal syndrome develops. Buspirone is rated Pregnancy Category B (see GLOSSARY; see also DRUG USE IN PREGNANCY/ LACTATION, page 162); data are lacking with regard to use in nursing mothers. Generally, avoid use in these patients.

Dosing Guidelines

Usual starting dose: 15 mg/d (7.5 mg BID) for 1 week; increase by 5 mg every few days as tolerated until a daily dose of 30 mg is reached. Do not exceed 60 mg/d. Although improvement will be noted within 2 weeks, optimal benefit may not be detected until 4 to 6 weeks of treatment.

MEPROBAMATE
Mechanism

Meprobamate interacts with, but does not bind per se to, the benzodiazepine-GABA-receptor complex.[263] Meprobamate causes sedation by inhibiting central adenosine reuptake and may reduce the increased norepinephrine turnover that occurs in response to stress. Meprobamate has mild muscle-relaxant and anticonvulsant properties.

Pharmacokinetics

Peak plasma meprobamate levels occur 1 to 3 hours after oral dosing. The drug is not highly protein bound (15%), and it is hepatically metabolized. The acute $t_{1/2}$ (6 to 17 h) increases with chronic use (24 to 48 h). Meprobamate may induce some hepatic enzymes, but little data are available.

Efficacy

Meprobamate has been available in the US for more than 40 years but well-designed efficacy studies are lacking. Although probably similar in efficacy to the benzodiazepines, meprobamate generally has been replaced by benzodiazepines or buspirone. It may be useful as a third- or fourth-line anxiolytic.[263] Use of meprobamate for more than 4 months is not recommended without periodic assessment of the need for anxiolytic therapy.

Drug Interactions

Patients taking meprobamate with alcohol, narcotics, barbiturates, or other CNS depressants may experience additive clinical effects; avoid these combinations.

Safety

Common side effects of meprobamate include drowsiness, ataxia, slurred speech, and weakness; paradoxical excitation with euphoria or overstimulation also may occur. Meprobamate may cause nausea, vomiting, diarrhea, palpitations, tachycardia, and transient ECG changes. Allergic or idiosyncratic hypersensitivity reactions ranging from mild localized erythematous rashes to bronchospasm, angioneurotic edema, and anaphylaxis may occur after only a few doses of meprobamate in patients who have never used the drug. Stevens-Johnson syndrome has occurred with meprobamate.

Meprobamate is a drug of abuse and it causes physical and psychological dependence. A Pregnancy Category rating has not been assigned for meprobamate, but this drug probably should be avoided in pregnancy (see also DRUG USE IN PREGNANCY/LACTATION, page 162). Meprobamate crosses the placental barrier and can cause congenital malformations during the first trimester. Meprobamate passes into breast milk at up to four times maternal plasma levels.

Warnings/Precautions

Meprobamate may precipitate seizures in epileptic patients and, like barbiturates, it is contraindicated in porphyria and in patients who exhibit sensitivity or allergy to it or to related compounds (eg, carisoprodol [Soma®]). Abrupt discontinuation after chronic use may precipitate a withdrawal syndrome; seizures may occur during withdrawal, especially in seizure-prone patients.

Dosing Guidelines

Usual starting dose: 1.2 to 1.6 g/d divided TID or QID. Do not exceed 2.4 g/d. A sustained-release product is available and can be given as 400 to 800 mg BID. Dosage reductions are not needed in renal or hepatic impairment, but observe patients for exaggerated clinical effects.

Sedative-Hypnotics

This section includes a discussion of barbiturates and miscellaneous nonbarbiturate sedative-hypnotics. Benzodiazepines used as sedative-hypnotics are discussed in the BENZODIAZEPINES section (page 113). The antihistamine diphenhydramine also is commonly used as a sedative-hypnotic (page 147).

BARBITURATES

Because they are safer and cause less dependency and less *hangover*, benzodiazepines have generally replaced barbiturates as sedative agents. Additionally, barbiturates often become ineffective after as few as 2 weeks of use as hypnotics. Nonetheless, this section provides a brief discussion of oral sedative-hypnotic barbiturate products including aprobarbital, butabarbital, mephobarbital, pentobarbital, phenobarbital, and secobarbital (Table 72). Anticonvulsant or anesthetic uses are not discussed.

Table 72. Overview of oral barbiturate therapy

Feature	Comments
Mechanism	Complex, not fully known; potentiates GABA transmission in brain. Enhances but does not displace benzodiazepine binding. ↓ Sleep latency (time to sleep onset); discontinuation → insomnia and ↑ REM sleep[266]
Pharmacokinetics	Rapid oral absorption on empty stomach; variable onset/duration of action (Table 73), extensive distribution, hepatic metabolism (inactive metabolites).[266] ↓ Metabolism in hepatic disease. May induce their own metabolism; many clinically important drug interactions
Efficacy	Largely replaced by benzodiazepines; efficacy ↓ after 2 weeks
Safety	Sedation, respiratory and cardiovascular depression. Consider tolerance, dependence, and abuse issues. Potentially lethal in overdose
Dosing	Individualize; use lowest effective dose for shortest possible duration (≤2 weeks for insomnia)

Abbreviations defined in GLOSSARY.

Table 73. Comparative pharmacokinetic features of oral barbiturate sedative-hypnotic drugs

Drug	Usual dose (mg/d) Sedative	Hypnotic	Mean $t_{1/2}$ (h)	Onset (min)	Duration (h)
LONG-ACTING					
Mephobarbital (Mebaral®)	32 - 200	—	34	30 - ≥60	10 - 16
Phenobarbital (various)	30 - 120	100 - 320	79	30 - ≥60	10 - 16
INTERMEDIATE					
Aprobarbital (Alurate®)	120	40 - 160	24	45 - 60	6 - 8
Butabarbital (Butisol®)	45 - 120	50 - 100	100	45 - 60	6 - 8
SHORT-ACTING					
Pentobarbital (Nembutal®)	40 - 120	100	22 - 50[a]	10 - 15	3 - 4
Secobarbital (Seconal®)	—	100	28	10 - 15	3 - 4

Abbreviations defined in GLOSSARY.

[a]Dose-dependent $t_{1/2}$ ranges from 22 h (100 mg) to 50 h (50 mg).

Information in this table obtained from *Physicians' Desk Reference, Facts and Comparisons*, or *AHFS Drug Information*. Please refer to those sources for current and additional prescribing information.

Efficacy

Barbiturates depress CNS, respiratory, and motor activity and produce mild sedation, hypnosis, and coma. They are rarely used for their sedative properties; benzodiazepines are preferred. Barbiturates are indicated for short-term treatment of insomnia, but tolerance to hypnotic effects usually occurs after several days of use.[266]

Drug Interactions

Because barbiturates can induce hepatic-metabolizing enzymes, drug interactions are common, and often clinically significant (Table 74). Most interactions have occurred with phenobarbital.

Table 74. Common drug interactions with barbiturates

Interacting drug	Effect of interaction
Acetaminophen	High, chronic barbiturate doses may ↑ risk of hepatotoxicity
Alcohol, antihistamines	↑ CNS depression, death
Anticoagulants	May ↑ anticoagulant metabolism: ↓ efficacy; monitor PT when adding or stopping barbiturate therapy
β-Blockers	May alter propranolol, metoprolol (but not timolol) pharmacokinetic parameters
Carbamazepine	↓ Carbamazepine levels: ↓ efficacy
Chloramphenicol	Chloramphenicol may ↓ phenobarbital metabolism; barbiturates may ↑ chloramphenicol metabolism
Clonazepam	↑ Clonazepam clearance: ↓ levels and ↓ efficacy
Corticosteroids	↑ Corticosteroid metabolism
Doxycycline	Phenobarbital ↓ levels; effect may persist for several weeks after barbiturate therapy stopped
Felodipine	↓ Felodipine levels
Fenoprofen	↓ Fenoprofen bioavailability
MAOIs	↑ CNS depression (sedation)
Metronidazole	↓ Efficacy of metronidazole
Narcotic analgesics	May ↑ CNS depressant effects of meperidine; may ↓ activity of methadone
Oral contraceptives	↓ Efficacy; use another form of birth control while on barbiturate therapy
Phenytoin	Unpredictable effects; monitor barbiturate and phenytoin levels often
Quinidine	↓ Quinidine levels; monitor levels
Rifampin	May ↑ barbiturate metabolism: ↓ efficacy
TCAs	↓ TCA levels; possible additive CNS depression
Theophylline	↓ Theophylline levels: ↓ efficacy; monitor theophylline levels
Valproic acid	May ↓ barbiturate metabolism: ↑ sedative effects
Verapamil	↑ Verapamil clearance

Abbreviations defined in GLOSSARY.

Information in this table obtained from *Physicians' Desk Reference, Facts and Comparisons,* or *AHFS Drug Information.* Please refer to those sources for current and additional prescribing information.

Psychopharmacologic Agents

Safety

Common side effects include sedation, ataxia, impaired mental performance, confusion, headache, and fever. Other important effects include bradycardia, hypoventilation, and hypotension. Serious and potentially (although rarely) fatal dermatologic reactions (eg, Stevens-Johnson syndrome, toxic epidermal necrolysis) may occur with phenobarbital use (see prescribing information for full disclosure). Megaloblastic anemia has been reported. Small amounts of barbiturates are excreted in breast milk; barbiturates are rated Pregnancy Category D (see GLOSSARY; see also DRUG USE IN PREGNANCY/LACTATION, page 162).

Warnings/Precautions

Barbiturates are contraindicated in patients with porphyria, severe liver or renal disease, or severe respiratory disease marked by dyspnea or obstruction (eg, sleep apnea). Because psychological and physical dependence and tolerance can occur (especially with high doses given chronically), administer barbiturates carefully, if at all, to anyone with a history of drug abuse or suicidal tendencies. The withdrawal syndrome includes anxiety, agitation, and possibly, seizures. Barbiturates may cause paradoxical excitation; the person may appear inebriated. Overdose causes fatal cardiovascular and respiratory depression. Successful suicide attempts have occurred with barbiturates alone or in combination with other drugs (eg, alcohol).

Dosing Guidelines

See prescribing information for specific dosing recommendations. Individualized dosing is important and use for more than 2 weeks is not recommended. Use low starting doses in elderly patients or those with hepatic or renal impairment. Serum-level monitoring is not required when barbiturates are used for short-term management of insomnia.

NONBARBITURATE HYPNOTICS

Therapeutic use of older nonbarbiturate hypnotics (eg, chloral hydrate or ethchlorvynol) has generally been replaced by safer and more effective agents (eg, benzodiazepines, zolpidem). However, clinicians may still see elderly patients who use these products for insomnia. A brief discussion of these older agents is followed by a thorough discussion of zolpidem, a highly effective and well-tolerated nonbenzodiazepine nonbarbiturate hypnotic agent.

Mechanism

The precise mechanism of action of the older nonbarbiturate hypnotics is not known. Chloral hydrate causes mild cerebral depression but little depression of respiration, BP, or reflexes.

Pharmacokinetics

Chloral hydrate is rapidly absorbed and metabolized to an active metabolite with a long $t_{1/2}$ (Table 75); this metabolite is subsequently converted to a highly protein-bound inactive by-product. Ethchlorvynol is rapidly absorbed and inactivated in the liver.

Table 75. Comparative pharmacokinetic features of older, oral nonbarbiturate hypnotics

Drug	Usual dose (mg/d)	Mean $t_{1/2}$ (h)	Onset (min)	Duration (h)
Chloral hydrate (Noctec®)	500 - 1000	7 - 10	30	NA
Ethchlorvynol (Placidyl®)	500	1 - 3 (acute) 10 - 20 (chronic)	15 - 60	5

NA = not available; other abbreviations defined in GLOSSARY.

Information in this table obtained from *Physicians' Desk Reference, Facts and Comparisons,* or *AHFS Drug Information.* Please refer to those sources for current and additional prescribing information.

Efficacy

Older nonbarbiturate hypnotics are indicated for short-term (<7 days) relief of insomnia. Chloral hydrate loses efficacy after about 2 weeks of use and ethchlorvynol after about 1 week.

Drug Interactions

A summary of drug interactions with the older nonbarbiturate hypnotics is provided in Table 76. Laboratory tests that may be altered by chloral hydrate include the copper sulfate test for glycosuria (glucose oxidase not affected) and fluorometric tests for urine catecholamines.

Table 76. Common drug interactions reported with older nonbarbiturate hypnotics

Interacting drug	Effect of interaction
Alcohol	↑ CNS depression. Avoid concurrent use with chloral hydrate because of mutual inhibition of metabolism and possible disulfiram-like reaction
Anticoagulants	Chloral hydrate may displace anticoagulant from protein-binding sites: ↑ anticoagulant response. Ethchlorvynol may ↓ anticoagulant response. Monitor PT and adjust dose if needed
Barbiturates	↑ CNS depression
Phenytoin	Chloral hydrate may ↑ phenytoin $t_{1/2}$: ↓ efficacy. Monitor levels

Abbreviations defined in GLOSSARY.

Information in this table obtained from *Physicians' Desk Reference, Facts and Comparisons,* or *AHFS Drug Information.* Please refer to those sources for current and additional prescribing information.

Safety

Common side effects of chloral hydrate include disorientation, somnambulism, incoherence, nausea, dyspepsia, hangover, and an unpleasant taste. Allergic skin rashes can occur. Gastrointestinal symptoms and skin rashes have occurred with ethchlorvynol. These products are rated Pregnancy Category C (see GLOSSARY; see also DRUG USE IN PREGNANCY/LACTATION, page 162) and should not be used by nursing mothers.

Warnings/Precautions

Avoid use of chloral hydrate in patients with esophagitis, gastritis, or ulcers. In patients with porphyria, use chloral hydrate carefully; ethchlorvynol is contraindicated. Chronic use of older nonbarbiturate hypnotics has been associated with abuse, tolerance, and physical dependence. Sudden discontinuation may cause a potentially fatal withdrawal syndrome. Overdose leads to respiratory depression and cardiovascular collapse.

Dosing Guidelines

Chloral hydrate: 500 mg to 1 g taken 15 to 30 minutes before bedtime with a full glass of water or juice to reduce stomach irritation; advise patient not to chew capsules. *Ethchlorvynol:* 500 mg HS; may increase to 750 mg if response inadequate. If patients experience early-morning awakening, a supplemental dose of 200 mg may be administered at that time.

ZOLPIDEM

Zolpidem tartrate (Ambien®) (Table 77) is the first of a new class of non-benzodiazepine nonbarbiturate hypnotic agents, the imidazopyridines. It is indicated for short-term treatment of insomnia.

Table 77. Overview of zolpidem therapy

Feature	Comments
Mechanism	Selective binding to central BZ_1 receptors ↑ GABA transmission → sedation. No binding to BZ_2 or BZ_3 receptors, so lacks anxiolytic, muscle relaxant, anticonvulsant activity[267]
Pharmacokinetics	Rapid sleep onset (15 - 20 min) may be delayed by food. 92% protein bound, extensive hepatic metabolism, ≥3 inactive by-products are renally eliminated. $t_{1/2}$ 1.5 - 3 h. Altered pharmacokinetics in elderly and renal or hepatic disease.[267] Drug interactions rare (except alcohol)
Efficacy	Highly effective quick-acting hypnotic for short-term treatment of insomnia
Safety	Well tolerated; drowsiness, dizziness, diarrhea common. No effect on sleep stages or REM sleep; no rebound insomnia, daytime hangover, or withdrawal syndrome. Some tolerance and dependence reported
Dosing	10 mg HS (elderly 5 mg HS). Do not exceed 10 mg HS

Abbreviations defined in GLOSSARY.

Efficacy

Highly sedating, zolpidem is an effective hypnotic.[262,267,268] Zolpidem does not alter sleep stages or REM sleep; it also does not appear to produce rebound insomnia, daytime hangover, or withdrawal effects. Tolerance to the hypnotic effects and dependence have been reported.[269,270] A 10-mg dose (5 mg in the elderly) is the most clinically effective; higher doses provide no significant clinical advantages but increase the side-effect profile.

Drug Interactions

Drug interactions (Table 78) are uncommon with zolpidem. Zolpidem pharmacokinetic parameters are not altered by alcohol, caffeine, haloperidol, chlorpromazine, cimetidine, ranitidine, warfarin, or digoxin.[267]

Table 78. Common drug interactions reported with zolpidem[267]

Interacting drug	Effect of interaction
Alcohol	↑ CNS depression
Cimetidine	↓ Alertness reported
Imipramine	↓ Imipramine levels; anterograde amnesia reported
Chlorpromazine	↑ Psychomotor impairment

Abbreviations defined in GLOSSARY.

Information in this table obtained from *Physicians' Desk Reference, Facts and Comparisons,* or *AHFS Drug Information.* Please refer to those sources for current and additional prescribing information.

Safety

With short-term use at recommended doses, the most common side effects are drowsiness, dizziness, and diarrhea. There is potential for dependence or abuse;[269] withdrawal symptoms are uncommon but have been reported when the drug is discontinued.[267,270] Zolpidem is rated Pregnancy Category B (see GLOSSARY; see also DRUG USE IN PREGNANCY/LACTATION, page 162). Although only small amounts (<.02%) of a dose are excreted in breast milk, use in nursing mothers is not recommended.

Warnings/Precautions

Use carefully in patients with reduced respiratory capacity because depression may occur. Administer cautiously in depressed patients, especially those who are suicidal. Although a withdrawal syndrome is unlikely, it has been reported and may include rebound insomnia, tremors, seizures, and agitation.[270] Observe patients discontinuing zolpidem therapy for nausea, flushing, fatigue, or nervousness as well as for more severe withdrawal symptoms.

Dosing Guidelines

Usual starting dose: 10 mg HS; higher doses do not offer greater efficacy. A dose of 5 mg HS is recommended for elderly patients (>65 y) or those with hepatic impairment; increase the dose to 10 mg only if needed. The maximum daily dose is 10 mg. Dosage adjustments are not needed for renally impaired patients, but monitor them for exaggerated clinical effects. For faster onset, advise patients to take on an empty stomach immediately before bedtime.

Antipsychotics

Antipsychotics are a large group of chemically distinct compounds with common beneficial and adverse pharmacologic effects (Table 79). Members of a subclass with similar side-chain substitution (eg, thioridazine, mesoridazine) tend to share certain pharmacologic effects (Table 80). The second-generation "atypical" antipsychotics (eg, clozapine, quetiapine, risperidone, and olanzapine) differ greatly in their neurotransmitter binding and side-effect profiles as compared with "typical" antipsychotics and are discussed separately (see page 136).

TYPICAL ANTIPSYCHOTICS

Because antipsychotics depress or reduce conditioned behavioral responses, emotional display, level of initiative and interest, and auditory hallucinations and delusions, and induce generalized sedation, they are useful in treating psychotic disorders (eg, schizophrenia) and psychotic behavior (eg, as might occur in Alzheimer's disease [AD] or in the early stages of a manic episode). However, they are not universally effective, and significant side effects affect nearly every organ system and tend to limit patient compliance. Haloperidol is the prototype *high-potency* antipsychotic and chlorpromazine the *low-potency* antipsychotic (reviewed in references 204 and 209).

Table 79. Overview of "typical" antipsychotic drug therapy

Feature	Comments
Mechanism	Block postsynaptic DA (D_1, D_2, D_3, D_4) receptors. Some also act as antagonists at α_1-adrenergic, serotonergic, histaminergic, and cholinergic receptors
Pharmacokinetics[a]	Variable oral absorption (oral liquids absorbed faster and more predictably than oral solid dosage forms), ≥90% protein bound, lipophilic (readily enter CNS), extensive hepatic metabolism with potentially active metabolites. $t_{1/2}$ ≤30 h. Drug interactions common
Efficacy	↓ Hallucinations, delusions, disorganized thoughts, but generally do not relieve blunted affect, withdrawal, and apathy
Safety	Drowsiness, anticholinergic-related effects, cardiac effects, photosensitivity. Serious: EPS and TD (common), NMS and ↓ WBC (rare)
Dosing	Individualize; ↑ gradually, do not adjust more than weekly. Full clinical benefit in ≥6 weeks

Abbreviations defined in GLOSSARY.

[a]Oral antipsychotics only. Use injectable dosage forms for rapid symptomatic relief. Long-acting (depot) intramuscular (IM) dosage forms also are available (eg, fluphenazine enanthate, fluphenazine decanoate, haloperidol decanoate).

Table 80. Comparative features of typical oral antipsychotics[209]

Drug	Equipotent dose[a] (mg)	Usual dose range (mg/d)	Sedation	EPS	Anticholinergic	Orthostatic hypotension
Chlorpromazine[b] (Thorazine®)	100	200 - 800	+++	++	++	+++
Thioridazine[c] (Mellaril®)	100	150 - 800	+++	+	+++	+++
Mesoridazine[c] (Serentil®)	50	30 - 400	+++	+	+++	++
Fluphenazine[d] (Prolixin®)	2	0.5 - 40	+	+++	+	+
Perphenazine[d] (Trilafon®)	10	8 - 64	+	+++	+	+
Prochlorperazine[d] (Compazine®)	15	15 - 150	++	+++	+	+
Trifluoperazine[d] (Stelazine®)	5	2 - 40	+	+++	+	+
Thiothixene[e] (Navane®)	4	5 - 30	+	+++	+	+
Haloperidol (Haldol®)	2	2 - 20	+	+++	+	+
Molindone (Moban®)	10	15 - 225	+	+++	+	+
Loxapine (Loxitane®)	15	20 - 250	++	+++	+	++

+++ = high; ++ = moderate; + = low; other abbreviations defined in GLOSSARY.

[a]Approximate dose equivalency. [b]An aliphatic phenothiazine. [c]A piperidine phenothiazine. [d]A piperazine phenothiazine. [e]A thioxanthene.

Information in this table obtained from Physicians' Desk Reference, Facts and Comparisons, or AHFS Drug Information. Please refer to those sources for current and additional prescribing information.

Efficacy

Antipsychotic drugs have been well studied, and they are all similarly effective for the treatment of psychotic disorders.[203] Primary differences are in the type and severity of side effects and drug interactions. A patient who fails to respond to one antipsychotic may respond to one from a different class. These drugs tend to be more effective in resolving hallucinations, delusions, and disorganized thoughts (positive symptoms) than in relieving blunted affect, emotional withdrawal, and lack of interest (negative symptoms).[271] Negative symptoms often mimic common antipsychotic side effects, making determination of therapeutic benefit difficult. In contrast, newer atypical antipsychotics (see page 136) relieve both positive and negative psychotic symptoms.

Drug Interactions

Drugs may either compete with antipsychotics for hepatic enzyme-binding sites (which would increase antipsychotic plasma levels) or enhance their metabolism (which would decrease plasma levels) (Table 81). Antipsychotics may cause false-positive laboratory tests (eg, urobilinogen, amylase, phenylketonuria, pregnancy tests, etc).

Table 81. Common drug interactions with typical antipsychotics

Interacting drug	Effect of interaction
Alcohol, CNS depressants	↑ CNS depression, ↑ EPS
Aluminum-containing antacids	↓ GI absorption: ↓ efficacy; administer 1 - 2 h apart
Anticholinergics	↓ Efficacy and worsening of psychotic symptoms; ↑ anticholinergic side effects
Barbiturates	Barbiturates ↑ antipsychotic metabolism: ↓ levels, ↓ efficacy. Also ↓ barbiturate levels
Bromocriptine	↓ Bromocriptine efficacy (phenothiazine)
Carbamazepine	↓ Haloperidol levels: ↓ efficacy
Epinephrine	Chlorpromazine may reverse/blunt pressor effect
Fluvoxamine	Fluvoxamine may ↓ metabolism: ↑ haloperidol levels; severe EPS reported
Lithium	Phenothiazines or haloperidol may ↑ disorientation, neurotoxicity, EPS
Meperidine	Phenothiazines may ↑ sedation and hypotension
Phenytoin	↑ Or ↓ phenytoin levels; ↓ haloperidol levels
Propranolol	↑ Propranolol and phenothiazine levels; may cause hypotension
TCA	Phenothiazines or haloperidol may ↑ TCA levels; TCA also may ↑ antipsychotic levels
Valproic acid	Chlorpromazine may ↑ valproic acid trough levels and $t_{1/2}$

Abbreviations defined in GLOSSARY.

Information in this table obtained from *Physicians' Desk Reference, Facts and Comparisons,* or *AHFS Drug Information.* Please refer to those sources for current and additional prescribing information.

Safety

Side effects can broadly be grouped into four categories: sedation, EPS, anticholinergic effects, and antiadrenergic effects (orthostatic hypotension) (see Table 80). Although certain subclasses are more likely than others to cause some side effects (Table 82), the potential exists for any adverse event to occur with any antipsychotic in a given patient. Refer to prescribing information for specific safety data (also see reference 203 for comprehensive summary).

Table 82. Broad safety differences between antipsychotic subclasses

Subclass (prototype)	More likely to cause	Less likely to cause
Aliphatic (chlorpromazine)	Sedation, hypotension, dermatitis, convulsions	EPS
Piperazine (fluphenazine)	EPS	Sedation, hypotension, retinal toxicity
Piperidine (thioridazine)	Retinal toxicity (at doses >800 mg/d), ejaculatory disturbances, ECG changes	EPS
Thioxanthene (thiothixene)	Sedation, EPS	Sedation (thiothixene), anticholinergic effects, hypotension
Butyrophenone (haloperidol)	EPS	Sedation, anticholinergic effects, hypotension

Abbreviations defined in GLOSSARY.

Information in this table obtained from *Physicians' Desk Reference, Facts and Comparisons*, or *AHFS Drug Information*. Please refer to those sources for current and additional prescribing information.

Drowsiness is common during the first 2 weeks of treatment, but tolerance usually develops to this side effect. Reduce the dose if drowsiness is excessive or persistent. Other common side effects include increased pulse rate, pruritus, dry mouth, nasal congestion, nausea, constipation; photosensitivity reactions can develop during chronic, high-dose therapy. Menstrual abnormalities and libido changes in women may be related to dopamine-receptor blockade and elevation of prolactin secretion or inhibition of gonadotropin release.[271] Erectile and ejaculatory dysfunction in men tends to be dose-related and more common with low-potency drugs (eg, chlorpromazine). Low-potency antipsychotics may prolong QT intervals.

Agranulocytosis is rare with typical antipsychotics but can develop after 4 to 10 weeks. Advise patients to report severe fever, sore mouth, gums, throat, and other signs of infection. Mild leukopenia does not require discontinuation of therapy. Tardive dyskinesia (TD; see GLOSSARY) is unpredictable and may be irreversible. Neuroleptic malignant syndrome (NMS; see GLOSSARY) is reported most often with haloperidol and depot (ie, intramuscular [IM]) antipsychotics, but has occurred with thiothixene, thioridazine, and virtually all antipsychotic drugs. Antipsychotics can suppress the cough reflex and, in elderly or lethargic patients, may decrease central thirst sensation, leading to hemoconcentration and dehydration. Rarely, fatal bronchopneumonia has resulted. Discontinue antipsychotic therapy if jaundice (hypersensitivity reaction presenting as a febrile, flu-like illness) occurs within 2 to 4 weeks after starting therapy.

Warnings/Precautions

Antipsychotics are contraindicated in patients with liver damage, severe hypotension or hypertension, bone marrow depression, or blood dyscrasias and should be used cautiously in selected patients (Table 83).

Table 83. Cautions related to antipsychotic drug use

Use with caution in	Comments
↑ QT interval	Low-potency drugs (eg, chlorpromazine) have quinidine-like activity
Parkinson's disease	↑ EPS
Glaucoma	Anticholinergic effects may cause blurry vision; lens deposits and opacities also reported
Seizure history	↓ Seizure threshold → grand or petit mal seizures. More common with ↑ sedating agents. Sudden death (brain-damaged or seizure patients taking ↑ doses) possible
Breast cancer	Persistent ↑ prolactin not known to be associated with breast cancer but caution advised
Renal impairment	Monitor renal function, ↓ dose if BUN ↑
Hepatic impairment	Encephalopathy may ↑ sensitivity to CNS effects; cholestatic jaundice (chlorpromazine) may ↓ drug clearance
Exposure to extremes of temperature	↓ Body temperature regulation; may cause hypothermia or hyperthermia

Abbreviations defined in GLOSSARY.

Information in this table obtained from *Physicians' Desk Reference, Facts and Comparisons,* or *AHFS Drug Information.* Please refer to those sources for current and additional prescribing information.

Avoid in nursing mothers; safety during pregnancy has not been established (see DRUG USE IN PREGNANCY/LACTATION, page 162). All agents have been reported to cross the placenta, and teratogenicity is not well studied; use in late trimesters may cause hypotension and EPS. Carefully consider the risk-to-benefit ratio before prescribing antipsychotics to pregnant women.

Use cautiously in depressed patients, particularly those who are suicidal. However, patients with psychotic depression require combination therapy with an antipsychotic and an antidepressant. An overdose presents as significant CNS depression (somnolence, deep sleep, or coma) with hypotension but also could present as agitation/restlessness, convulsions, fever, and ECG changes; EPS also may occur. Hospitalize patients who have overdosed for supportive measures.

Dosing Guidelines

There is a wide range of effective doses for antipsychotic drugs. Refer to Table 80 or to prescribing information for guidance. In general, individualize doses, use the lowest effective dose, and increase doses slowly (not more than weekly). Administer one third to one fourth the usual adult dose in elderly or emaciated patients because they are more susceptible to both beneficial and adverse drug effects. Increase doses very slowly in these patients. It may take 6 weeks or more to see the full clinical benefit of antipsychotic therapy. Abrupt withdrawal of high-dose therapy may cause a syndrome of GI distress (diarrhea), dizziness, headache, tachycardia, insomnia, dyskinesia, and akathisia; gradual dose reduction is suggested. Use antipsychotics only if needed and at the lowest effective dose and in nonschizophrenic patients for the shortest possible time to maintain efficacy and minimize toxicity.

Use divided doses initially but consider HS dosing when an effective dosage is achieved because of the long duration of therapeutic effect. A correlation between clinical effect and plasma level has been demonstrated for some antipsychotics but remains controversial.[272] Monitoring plasma levels may sometimes be useful to oversee patient compliance, avoid toxicity, and assess drug interactions.

ATYPICAL ANTIPSYCHOTICS

For some patients, atypical antipsychotics (eg, clozapine, olanzapine, quetiapine, and risperidone) offer significant efficacy and safety advantages over typical antipsychotics (Table 84). First, they cause minimal EPS, little to no TD, and minimal hyperprolactinemia at usual doses. Second, they tend to improve negative as well as positive symptoms of schizophrenia and are more likely to be effective in treatment-refractory patients (see page 73). Finally, as a class, they cause less cognitive impairment and may actually improve cognition (ie, diminished behavioral and emotional responses) and therefore are better tolerated. Many of these benefits are directly related to the different neurotransmitter receptor-binding profiles as compared with typical antipsychotics (see Mechanism below) (also see references 203 and 273 for comprehensive summaries).

Mechanism

Clozapine binds preferentially to serotonergic (5-HT$_2$) receptors followed by α_1-adrenergic, histaminergic (H$_1$), and muscarinic cholinergic receptors; it also blocks dopamine (D$_1$, D$_2$, and D$_4$) receptors. Olanzapine binds similarly to serotonergic, dopaminergic, histaminergic, α-adrenergic, and cholinergic receptors.

Risperidone blocks serotonergic receptors and has a high affinity for α-adrenergic, dopaminergic, and histaminergic receptors. It has little to no affinity for cholinergic or ß-adrenergic receptors. Quetiapine blocks 5-HT$_2$ receptors with a greater affinity than it does D$_2$ receptors; it also antagonizes histamine and/or α-adrenergic receptors but does not bind to cholinergic muscarinic or benzodiazepine receptors.[274-276]

Table 84. Overview of "atypical" antipsychotic drug therapy[277]

Drug	Usual dose range (mg/d)	Sedation	EPS	Anticholinergic	Orthostatic hypotension
Clozapine (Clozaril®)	300 - 900	+++	0/+	+++	+++
Olanzapine (Zyprexa®)	5 - 20	+	0/+	+/++	+
Quetiapine (Seroquel®)	150 - 600	+	0/+	0/+	+
Risperidone (Risperdal®)	1 - 6	+	0/+[a]	0/+	+

+++ = high; ++ = moderate; + = low; 0 = insignificant, similar to placebo; other abbreviations defined in GLOSSARY.

[a]Dose-related; greater at doses >6 mg/d.

Information in this table obtained from *Physicians' Desk Reference, Facts and Comparisons,* or *AHFS Drug Information.* Please refer to those sources for current and additional prescribing information.

CLOZAPINE

Clozapine was the first atypical antipsychotic marketed in the US. Although very effective, it is associated with severe, potentially fatal agranulocytosis in a small percentage of patients and thus is generally reserved for severely ill patients who do not respond to a treatment course (adequate dose, duration) with typical antipsychotics.

Pharmacokinetics

Oral clozapine is well absorbed; peak plasma levels occur within 6 hours (average 2.5 h). The drug can be taken without regard to meals. Clozapine is highly (95%) protein bound, and although drug interactions have not been fully evaluated (Table 85), monitor plasma levels of concurrently administered highly protein-bound drugs (eg, warfarin, phenytoin, digoxin) when clozapine therapy is started or stopped or when the dose is adjusted. Clozapine is almost completely metabolized, primarily by CYP1A2. One metabolite (norclozapine) may have therapeutic activity as well as toxic effects on hematopoietic precursors.[278] The long $t_{1/2}$ (10 to 17 h) permits HS dosing. Many SSRIs (eg, fluoxetine, paroxetine, fluvoxamine, and sertraline) increase plasma levels of clozapine and norclozapine.[226]

Table 85. Common drug interactions with clozapine[226,275,278,279]

Interacting drug	Effect of interaction
Cimetidine	↓ Clozapine metabolism: ↑ levels
Erythromycin	↓ Clozapine metabolism: ↑ levels
Ketoconazole	↓ Clozapine metabolism: ↑ levels
Phenytoin, carbamazepine	↑ Clozapine metabolism: ↓ levels (↑ risk of agranulocytosis with carbamazepine); monitor phenytoin levels
Risperidone	↑ Levels of clozapine and risperidone
SSRIs	↓ Clozapine metabolism: ↑ levels

Abbreviations defined in GLOSSARY.
Information in this table obtained from *Physicians' Desk Reference, Facts and Comparisons,* or *AHFS Drug Information*. Please refer to those sources for current and additional prescribing information.

Efficacy

Clozapine is significantly more effective than chlorpromazine in severe, chronic schizophrenia.[280,281] It also may improve cognitive functioning to a greater degree than typical antipsychotics.[210] A therapeutic plasma-level range has not been firmly established although levels of at least 350 mg/dL may predict response.[278] There is considerable evidence that clozapine is effective in the treatment of not only schizophrenia, but refractory mania as well.[282]

Safety

Common side effects include drowsiness and sedation, dizziness, vertigo, headache, hypersalivation, tachycardia, hypotension, constipation, and nausea. Transient, benign temperature elevation may occur in the first weeks of treatment; consider NMS or agranulocytosis (see Warnings/Precautions) in these patients. Significant weight gain occurs with long-term therapy and significantly interferes with compliance. Clozapine is rated Pregnancy Category B (see GLOSSARY; see also DRUG USE IN PREGNANCY/LACTATION, page 162); do not give to nursing mothers. Clozapine causes few EPS and little or no elevation in plasma prolactin levels. The possibility, although rare, exists that either TD or NMS could develop with clozapine.[283]

Warnings/Precautions

Clozapine carries a significant risk (cumulative incidence at 1 year of 1.3%) of potentially life-threatening agranulocytosis (WBC <500/mm³). Elderly patients and women may be at greater risk, and a disproportionate number of cases have occurred in patients of Jewish background. A baseline WBC count with differential and weekly WBC monitoring is required for the duration of therapy and for 4 weeks after the drug is discontinued. The *Clozaril®* Patient *Management System* links WBC testing (see current prescribing information for specific WBC monitoring guidelines), patient monitoring, and pharmacy distribution services to compliance with safety monitoring. Patients cannot receive more than a 1-week supply. Clozapine is contraindicated in patients with myeloproliferative disorders or a history of clozapine-induced agranulocytosis or severe granulocytopenia, or in anyone receiving myelosuppressive therapy. It should never be prescribed concurrently with carbamazepine because of its additive bone marrow toxicity.

Clozapine may increase seizure activity (cumulative incidence at 1 year of 5%) in a dose-related manner (1% at <300 mg/d and 4.4% at >600 mg/d).[277] Administer carefully to patients with a seizure history or those taking drugs with increased seizure potential (eg, bupropion, maprotiline). Clozapine may potentiate the pharmacologic effects of anticholinergic, antihypertensive, and CNS-depressant drugs (eg, alcohol, benzodiazepines). Use clozapine carefully in patients with benign prostatic hypertrophy (BPH) or narrow-angle glaucoma (see Table 83). Limited data are available on clozapine use in patients with liver or renal impairment or cardiac disease.

Dosing Guidelines

Usual starting dose: 12.5 mg QD or BID; increase by 25 to 50 mg/d, if tolerated. The target dose is 300 to 450 mg/d at the end of 2 or 3 weeks. Make subsequent dose increases not more than weekly in increments of 100 mg or less. Plasma levels may be checked when the dose is stabilized. Slow dose titration may lower the risk of seizures, hypotension, and sedation. Clinical response is common at doses of 300 to 600 mg/d although higher doses are sometimes required. In patients taking doses of 550 mg/d or higher, concomitant use of an anticonvulsant is recommended to reduce seizure risk.

OLANZAPINE

Olanzapine is structurally similar to clozapine.

Pharmacokinetics

Olanzapine is well absorbed orally (more predictably than clozapine); peak levels occur within 6 hours. Food does not affect its absorption. Olanzapine is highly protein bound (93%) and undergoes extensive hepatic metabolism, primarily by CYP1A2; none of the metabolites has therapeutic activity. Clinically significant drug interactions have been reported (Table 86). QD dosing is appropriate in view of its 30-hour $t_{1/2}$. Because olanzapine is highly metabolized, hepatic but not renal disease may increase plasma levels. Gender differences are apparent (higher plasma levels in women due to lower clearance) but clinically unimportant. Smokers have a 40% to 50% higher clearance rate, and Japanese subjects may have longer $t_{1/2}$s.[279,284]

Table 86. Common drug interactions with olanzapine[279]

Interacting drug	Effect of interaction
Alcohol, CNS depressants	↑ Effects, use cautiously
Fluvoxamine	↓ Olanzapine metabolism: ↑ levels
Omeprazole	↑ Olanzapine metabolism: ↓ levels
Phenytoin, carbamazepine	Moderate ↓ olanzapine levels via ↑ metabolism; probably clinically irrelevant
Rifampin	↑ Olanzapine metabolism: ↓ levels

Abbreviations defined in GLOSSARY.

Information in this table obtained from *Physicians' Desk Reference, Facts and Comparisons,* or *AHFS Drug Information.* Please refer to those sources for current and additional prescribing information.

Efficacy

Clinical experience with olanzapine is limited but growing rapidly. In chronic schizophrenia, the drug is as effective as haloperidol and risperidone but causes less EPS and TD than the former.[284-286] There is a suggestion that the drug may produce a more robust response than other agents in some patients.

Safety

Olanzapine is generally well tolerated. Common side effects include somnolence, constipation, akathisia, headache, and weight gain.[284] The last side effect is problematic and associated with poor patient compliance. Cardiac manifestations (eg, orthostatic hypotension, dizziness, and tachycardia) are common but can be minimized by using a low starting dose with gradual upward titration. The development of EPS is not clinically important at doses less than 10 to 15 mg/d.[287] In spite of its chemical similarity to clozapine, olanzapine appears to be free from serious hematologic toxicity. It does not cause TD. However, as with all antipsychotics, if signs or symptoms of NMS or TD appear, discontinue the drug.

Warnings/Precautions

Use olanzapine cautiously in patients who have an underlying cardiac condition that would predispose to hypotensive episodes (eg, dehydration, antihypertensive medications). Use cautiously in patients taking CNS depressants (eg, alcohol, benzodiazepines). Many of the same precautions that apply to typical antipsychotics also apply to olanzapine (see Table 83), especially regarding modest, persistent hyperprolactinemia (at higher doses); use in patients with glaucoma, BPH, seizure history; and use in patients exposed to extremes of temperature. Olanzapine is rated Pregnancy Category C (see GLOSSARY; see also DRUG USE IN PREGNANCY/LACTATION, page 162) and should be avoided in nursing mothers. Use olanzapine cautiously in patients with liver dysfunction; periodic monitoring of transaminases is suggested in this population.

Dosing Guidelines

Usual starting dose: 5 to 10 mg HS (without regard to meals); increase to 10 mg HS after several days. Make subsequent dose adjustments (5 mg HS) not more than weekly because of the long $t_{1/2}$. The usual maximum dose is 20 mg/d. Some patients, however, require 30- to 40-mg daily doses. In the elderly or patients prone to hypotension, start with 2.5 to 5 mg QD and titrate more gradually. Dose adjustments are not needed in renally impaired patients.

QUETIAPINE

Quetiapine is the newest atypical antipsychotic to reach the US market. It is structurally related to clozapine and olanzapine. Like the other members of the class, it is less likely to cause EPS than typical antipsychotics.

Pharmacokinetics

Quetiapine is rapidly and completely absorbed after oral administration; it is metabolized via CYP3A4 to mostly inactive metabolites. The $t_{1/2}$ is 3 to 6 hours.[273,274] Drug interactions have not been fully evaluated but some clinically important interactions have been reported (Table 87). Other interactions related to inhibition of quetiapine metabolism via CYP3A4 have been postulated.

Table 87. Common drug interactions with quetiapine[274]

Interacting drug	Effect of interaction
Carbamazepine	May ↑ metabolism: ↓ levels
Erythromycin	Possible ↓ metabolism: ↑ levels, side effects
Fluvoxamine	Possible ↓ metabolism: ↑ levels, side effects
Ketoconazole	Possible ↓ metabolism: ↑ levels, side effects
Nefazodone	Possible ↓ metabolism: ↑ levels, side effects
Phenytoin	↑ Quetiapine clearance: marked ↓ levels
Thioridazine	May ↑ quetiapine clearance: ↓ levels

Information in this table obtained from *Physicians' Desk Reference, Facts and Comparisons,* or *AHFS Drug Information.* Please refer to those sources for current and additional prescribing information.

Efficacy

High-dose quetiapine (≤750 mg/d) was more effective than low-dose (≤250 mg/d) or placebo in treating schizophrenic patients in one 6-week trial.[288] Positive symptoms were consistently alleviated; negative symptoms, less so. Neither long-term efficacy nor comparative efficacy with other atypical antipsychotics has been evaluated to date.

Safety

Quetiapine is well tolerated; weight gain is a common side effect. Other side effects reported include somnolence, dizziness, constipation, postural hypotension, and dry mouth. Increased LFTs to three times the upper limit of normal have been reported usually within the first 3 weeks of treatment with quetiapine and have returned to baseline with continued treatment. Elevated cholesterol and triglyceride levels have been reported in patients taking quetiapine. Orthostatic hypotension can be minimized by starting with a low dose (25 mg BID) and increasing slowly. Tardive dyskinesia has occurred only rarely in patients also taking other antipsychotic drugs. Hyperprolactinemia does not appear to be a problem.[273,274]

Warnings/Precautions

Cataracts have occurred in dogs taking the drug chronically but have not been observed in human trials. A baseline slit-lamp exam is recommended and should be repeated every 6 months. One case of priapism has been reported with quetiapine. Quetiapine is not recommended for use by nursing women. General warnings and precautions are similar to those for other typical and atypical antipsychotic drugs.

Dosing Guidelines

Usual starting dose: 25 mg BID; increase by 25 or 50 mg BID or TID as tolerated after 2 or 3 days. Target range is 300 to 400 mg/d. Further dose increases if needed should occur at least 2 days apart. Slower titration and lower maintenance doses may be needed in the elderly or in patients with hepatic impairment because quetiapine is extensively metabolized.

Psychopharmacologic Agents

RISPERIDONE

Risperidone is structurally distinct from clozapine and olanzapine.

Pharmacokinetics

The absorption of risperidone is nearly complete and unaffected by food; peak plasma levels occur within 1 hour. Risperidone is extensively metabolized, primarily by CYP2D6, and one metabolite (9-hydroxy-risperidone) has therapeutic activity similar to the parent drug. A small percentage (<10%) of patients are genetically slow metabolizers of risperidone and may exhibit an increased response due to higher plasma levels. The overall mean $t_{1/2}$ is about 20 hours (parent and metabolite). Risperidone and 9-hydroxy-risperidone are 90% and 77% protein bound, respectively. Clearance of risperidone and its metabolite decreases by about 60% in patients with moderate to severe renal disease.

Drug Interactions

Clinically significant interactions have not been reported. Nonetheless, drugs that inhibit the CYP2D6 system could interfere with risperidone metabolism. Monitor patients closely for toxicity when such drugs (eg, SSRIs, TCAs) are added or removed from a therapeutic regimen.

Efficacy

The efficacy of risperidone has been demonstrated in short- and long-term (up to 12-month) trials of chronic schizophrenia. Risperidone is as effective as haloperidol but reportedly has a faster onset of action, a lower incidence of EPS, and more benefit on negative psychotic symptoms (see page 68).

Safety

Commonly reported side effects are sedation, EPS (dose-related), constipation, orthostatic dizziness, rhinitis, dyspepsia, and tachycardia. EPS occur at an incidence similar to placebo at doses of 4 to 6 mg/d, although some have argued that the rates of EPS on placebo in clinical trials were relatively high, suggesting carry-over effects from previous antipsychotics. TD is rare but should be considered if symptoms occur. Weight gain is not usual, but can be significant in a small percentage of patients, and is dose-related. Dermatologic reactions including photosensitivity are common; advise patients to use sunscreens and protective clothing. Risperidone is rated Pregnancy Category C (see GLOSSARY; see also DRUG USE IN PREGNANCY/LACTATION, page 162) and should not be used in nursing mothers.

Warnings/Precautions

Risperidone may potentiate the pharmacologic effects of antihypertensive agents and CNS depressants (eg, alcohol, benzodiazepines) and antagonize the effects of dopamine agonists (eg, levodopa). Persistent hyperprolactinemia has been reported; caution is advised in patients with a history of breast cancer (see Table 83). One case each of priapism (after 11 months of treatment) and thrombotic thrombocytopenic purpura has developed. Use cautiously in patients with a seizure history or those exposed to extremes of temperature.

Dosing Guidelines

Usual starting dose: 1 mg BID (0.5 mg BID in the elderly); increase by 1 mg BID (0.5 mg BID in the elderly) on days 2 and 3 if tolerated. The target dose after 3 days is 3 mg BID. This titration schedule using divided doses is suggested to minimize the risk of orthostatic hypotension. Make subsequent dose adjustments (1 mg BID) not less than weekly to permit a new steady-state level to be achieved. The dosage range is 4 to 16 mg/d, but optimal efficacy usually occurs at doses between 4 and 6 mg/d. Doses higher than 6 to 10 mg/d are usually not more effective and are associated with greater EPS, although these side effects may occur at lower doses also, particularly in the elderly. Restarting risperidone therapy in a patient who has been off the drug should be done using the 3-day titration schedule described above.

Usual starting dose in the elderly, in patients with severe renal (CrCl <30 mL/min) or hepatic disease, or in those at risk for hypotension: 0.5 mg BID; increase by 0.5 mg BID to the maximum dose of 4 mg/d.[289]

Drugs for Extrapyramidal Side Effects

EPS (see GLOSSARY) are a troublesome complication of typical antipsychotic drugs which, if misdiagnosed, could lead the physician to increase the antipsychotic dose that caused them in the first place. Antipsychotic drug-induced EPS are believed to result from blockade of dopaminergic receptors and the ensuing imbalance is manifested as a relative increase in cholinergic activity. Drug-induced EPS can be classified as acute dystonic reactions (eg, facial grimacing, oculogyric crisis, laryngospasm), akathisia (ie, subjective feeling of restlessness and objective restless movement), pseudoparkinson features (eg, slowed movement, masked facies, rigidity), and TD (ie, irregular oral, buccal, and facial movements). EPS, which may be severe, contribute to poor outcome by reducing patient compliance with therapy and exacerbating psychotic symptoms.[290] Although drug-induced EPS may be dose related and some antipsychotics may be less likely than others to cause the syndrome (see Table 80), symptoms require treatment in most cases. Agents used to manage drug-induced EPS include those that block or decrease cholinergic activity (eg, anticholinergics, antihistamines) or increase dopaminergic activity (eg, dopaminergics); ß-blockers and benzodiazepines also have been used with some success in akathisia.

ANTICHOLINERGICS

Oral anticholinergic drugs used to manage EPS include benztropine (Cogentin®), biperiden (Akineton®), procyclidine (Kemadrin®), and trihexyphenidyl (Artane®) (Table 88). Biperiden and procyclidine are trihexyphenidyl analogues.

Table 88. Overview of anticholinergic drugs for EPS

Feature	Comments
Mechanism	Block relative ↑ in cholinergic activity caused by antipsychotic drug-induced blockade of DA receptors
Pharmacokinetics	Little data. Peak levels usually within 1.5 h. Drug interactions with phenothiazines, DA agonists
Efficacy	↓ Rigidity, drooling, akinesia, and laryngospasm associated with acute EPS. Not effective in TD
Safety	Dry mouth (may be severe), rash, agitation, drowsiness, constipation, blurry vision, difficult urination. Elderly particularly sensitive and may become confused, disoriented, or psychotic. May unmask early Alzheimer's disease
Dosing	Individualize based on severity of EPS. Younger patients need and tolerate higher doses than the elderly. Take with meals to ↓ GI upset or before meals to ↓ dry mouth

Abbreviations defined in GLOSSARY.

Efficacy

Anticholinergic drugs reduce the severity of certain Parkinson-like symptoms (eg, tremor, drooling, rigidity, akinesia). TD (see GLOSSARY) is not responsive to anticholinergic therapy. Once EPS are controlled, therapy may be stopped without recurrence of EPS[291] but generally not if antipsychotic therapy is being continued.

Drug Interactions

Drug interactions involving anticholinergic agents used for EPS are shown in Table 89.

Table 89. Common drug interactions with anticholinergics used for EPS[290]

Interacting drug	Effect of interaction
Alcohol, CNS depressants	↑ CNS effects with anticholinergics; use cautiously
Amantadine	↑ Anticholinergic side effects
Digoxin	↑ Digoxin levels
Levodopa	Unresolved; ↓ GI motility from anticholinergics may ↑ gastric deactivation of levodopa: ↓ levodopa efficacy
TCAs	↑ Anticholinergic side effects

Abbreviations defined in GLOSSARY.

Information in this table obtained from *Physicians' Desk Reference, Facts and Comparisons*, or *AHFS Drug Information*. Please refer to those sources for current and additional prescribing information.

Safety

Common anticholinergic (atropine-like) side effects include dry mouth, GI upset, skin rash, CNS confusion, disorientation and agitation (delirium), drowsiness, hypotension, mild bradycardia, constipation, blurry vision, muscular weakness, difficult urination, decreased sweating, and erectile dysfunction. These drugs are rated Pregnancy Category C (see GLOSSARY; see also DRUG USE IN PREGNANCY/LACTATION, page 162); safety has not been established in nursing mothers and these agents may inhibit lactation.

Warnings/Precautions

Anticholinergics are contraindicated in angle-closure glaucoma, GI obstruction, megacolon, myasthenia gravis, BPH, or stenosing peptic ulcers. The elderly are particularly sensitive to anticholinergic side effects and may develop mental confusion, disorientation, hallucinations, or psychotic-like symptoms. Use cautiously in patients with cardiovascular conditions (eg, tachycardia, arrhythmias, hypertension, or hypotension). In hot weather, the elderly, alcoholic individuals, persons with CNS disease, or those who work in hot environments may be susceptible to the effects of anticholinergics; severe anhidrosis and fatal hyperthermia have occurred. Severe dry mouth requiring discontinuation of therapy may develop. Up to one third of patients who use anticholinergics may develop depression, confusion, hallucinations, or delusions. These are generally dose-related.

Dosing Guidelines

A flexible, individualized, and empiric dosing approach is needed based on the severity of the EPS. Younger patients require and tolerate higher doses than elderly patients. Take with meals to reduce GI upset or before meals to minimize dry mouth.

Trihexyphenidyl: Usual starting dose: 1 mg/d. If EPS are not controlled in a few hours, increase subsequent doses. Usual range is 5 to 15 mg/d divided QD or BID. If EPS are controlled for several days, it may be possible to reduce the dose or stop therapy without a symptomatic recurrence.[291] Do not use sustained-release product for initial therapy.

Benztropine: Usual starting dose: 1 to 4 mg QD or BID; individualize dose according to patient's need. In high doses (15 to 30 mg/d), benztropine may cause weakness and an inability to move certain muscle groups.

Procyclidine: Usual starting dose: 2.5 mg TID; increase by 2.5 mg/d until EPS relieved. Usual dosage range is 10 to 20 mg/d QD, BID, or TID.

Biperiden: Usual dose: 2 mg QD to TID.

ANTIHISTAMINES

Antihistamines with central anticholinergic activity (eg, diphenhydramine [Benadryl®]; Table 90) are effective for drug-induced EPS, whereas nonsedating antihistamines that do not penetrate the CNS (eg, astemizole, fexofenadine) are not.

Efficacy

Although less effective than anticholinergic agents for reducing the rigidity and involuntary movement of drug-induced EPS, diphenhydramine may be better tolerated, especially by the elderly.

Drug Interactions

Drug interactions reported with diphenhydramine are shown in Table 91.

Safety

The most common side effect is sedation, which can be mild or may cause deep sleep. Some individuals develop tolerance to this effect after several days. Diphenhydramine is more sedating than anticholinergic drugs, but this may be a useful feature in patients in whom akathisia is prominent. Anticholinergic side effects such as dry mouth, urinary retention, vertigo, blurry vision, and insomnia may occur. Nausea, anorexia, diarrhea, or constipation may develop. Cardiac side effects are infrequent in usual therapeutic doses. Safe use in pregnancy has not been established; diphenhydramine crosses the placenta and passes into breast milk and probably should be avoided in nursing mothers (see DRUG USE IN PREGNANCY/LACTATION, page 162).

Table 90. Overview of diphenhydramine for drug-induced EPS

Feature	Comments
Mechanism	Reversible histamine (H_1) blocker with substantial central anticholinergic (atropine-like) activity because of structural similarities with anticholinergics
Pharmacokinetics	Good oral absorption, peak effects 2 - 4 h after dosing, 85% protein bound; $t_{1/2}$ 3 - 9 h. Widely distributed (including CNS), nearly complete hepatic metabolism
Efficacy	Less effective than anticholinergics for ↓ rigidity and involuntary movement, but better tolerated, especially by the elderly
Safety	Sedation (mild to deep sleep; tolerance may develop), dry mouth, urinary retention, vertigo, blurry vision, insomnia
Dosing	25 - 50 mg TID or QID with meals to ↓ GI upset. Also, 10 - 50 mg deep IM used for acute dystonia

Abbreviations defined in GLOSSARY.

Table 91. Common drug interactions with diphenhydramine

Interacting drug	Effect of interaction
Alcohol, CNS depressants	↑ Sedative effects; use cautiously
MAOIs	May prolong and ↑ anticholinergic effects of antihistamines

Abbreviations defined in GLOSSARY.

Information in this table obtained from *Physicians' Desk Reference, Facts and Comparisons,* or *AHFS Drug Information.* Please refer to those sources for current and additional prescribing information.

Warnings/Precautions

Because it has significant anticholinergic activity, use diphenhydramine carefully in patients with angle-closure glaucoma, BPH, or GI obstruction (also see Warnings/Precautions for Anticholinergics, page 146). Epileptiform seizures may be precipitated in patients with focal lesions of the cerebral cortex; use the drug carefully in such patients.

Dosing Guidelines

Usual dose: 25 to 50 mg TID to QID taken with meals to reduce GI upset. For acute dystonia, use 10 to 50 mg deep IM.

DOPAMINERGICS

Among available dopaminergic agents, only the antiviral amantadine (Symmetrel®) is effective for drug-induced EPS (Table 92).

Table 92. Overview of amantadine therapy for EPS

Feature	Comments
Mechanism	Mechanism in drug-induced EPS unknown; may ↑ DA release from central storage sites or ↑ central catecholamine release. No known anticholinergic activity
Pharmacokinetics	Slow but complete oral absorption. Peak levels in 2.5 - 4 h, $t_{1/2}$ 14 - 16 h, 67% protein bound. Renally eliminated mostly unchanged. Benefit correlated with plasma levels of 0.12 - 1.12 µg/mL
Efficacy	Effective but not better than anticholinergics
Safety	Nausea, dizziness, insomnia, CNS stimulation. Less constipation, dry mouth, somnolence than with anticholinergics. Side effects ↑ if plasma levels >1.5 µg/mL (ie, elderly, renal impairment)
Dosing	Initial dose: 100 mg BID. Clinical benefit evident within 48 h, maximal in 2 weeks, and may ↓ after 4 weeks. ↑ To 300 mg/d (divided) if response not optimal. ↓ Dose in renal impairment and in patients >65 years of age (Table 93)

Abbreviations defined in GLOSSARY.

Efficacy

Amantadine is effective but not more efficacious than anticholinergic agents for drug-induced EPS. A maximal effect is usually seen in 2 weeks; efficacy may decline after 4 weeks.[290] Long-term efficacy data are unavailable.

Drug Interactions

Few interactions occur with amantadine. When used with an anticholinergic, the degree of anticholinergic side effects may be increased (see Table 89). Elevated plasma amantadine levels occurred in an elderly man taking a combination diuretic (triamterene/hydrochlorothiazide) concurrently.

Safety

Common side effects include nausea, dizziness, and insomnia. Less common are those related to CNS stimulation (eg, irritability, tremor, ataxia, agitation, reduced concentration). Anticholinergic-like effects (eg, constipation, dry mouth, somnolence) are observed but occur less frequently with amantadine than with anticholinergic drugs. Side effects of amantadine may be more common when plasma levels are higher than 1.5 µg/mL, which may occur more readily in the elderly or renally impaired patients. Amantadine is rated Pregnancy Category C (see GLOSSARY; see also DRUG USE IN PREGNANCY/LACTATION, page 162); it is excreted in breast milk.

Warnings/Precautions

Deaths have occurred with amantadine overdose, possibly because of cardiac arrhythmia, tachycardia, or hypertension. Suicide and suicide attempts also have occurred; the basis for this is unknown. Amantadine may exacerbate psychotic symptoms in patients with a history of mental disorders. Amantadine may increase seizure activity. Use cautiously in patients with CHF because amantadine induces catecholamine release.

Dosing Guidelines

Usual dose: 100 mg BID. Clinical benefit is evident within 48 hours and maximal effects within 2 weeks. Increase the dose to 300 mg/d (divided) if response is not optimal. Reduce the dose in renal impairment (Table 93).

Table 93. Dosing schedule for amantadine in renal impairment

CrCl (mL/min)	Amantadine dosage
30 - 50	200 mg on day 1 then 100 mg QD
15 - 29	200 mg on day 1 then 100 mg QOD
<15-hemodialysis	200 mg once weekly

Abbreviations defined in GLOSSARY.

Information in this table obtained from *Physicians' Desk Reference, Facts and Comparisons,* or *AHFS Drug Information.* Please refer to those sources for current and additional prescribing information.

ß-BLOCKERS

ß-Blockers are not indicated per se for treatment of drug-induced EPS, although propranolol, which is indicated for familial essential tremor, may be helpful. However, highly lipid-soluble (lipophilic) agents (eg, propranolol, pindolol, betaxolol) that cross the blood-brain barrier may improve EPS in some patients; these drugs may be most useful for the akathisia component of EPS.[292] Propranolol is the best studied of the class; it is fairly well tolerated in low doses (30 mg/d). The TCAs, antipsychotics, and SSRIs may decrease hepatic metabolism of ß-blockers and increase plasma levels of these drugs.

Cognitive Enhancers

ERGOLOID MESYLATES

Ergoloid mesylates (Hydergine®; dihydroergotoxine, dihydrogenated ergot alkaloids) are indicated for symptomatic relief of age-related mental capacity decline (in persons >60 years of age), such as that which might occur in AD (Table 94).

Table 94. Overview of ergoloid mesylate therapy

Feature	Comments
Mechanism	Exact mechanism unknown; may ↑ cerebral blood flow. Does not have vasoconstrictive properties like natural ergot alkaloids
Pharmacokinetics	Rapid oral absorption, extensive hepatic metabolism, drug interactions not reported
Efficacy	Modest ↑ in cognition at best
Safety	Transient nausea, GI disturbances
Dosing	1 mg TID; ↑ to 12 mg/d (divided); response usually requires ≥6 mg/d for 6 months

Abbreviations defined in GLOSSARY.

Efficacy

In 12-week studies using the Sandoz Clinical Assessment Geriatric Rating Scale, modest clinical but statistically significant improvements have been observed in mental alertness, confusion, orientation, emotional lability, recent memory, self-care, depression, anxiety, cooperation, sociability, appetite, dizziness, fatigue, and overall improvement in clinical status.

Safety

Ergoloid mesylates are generally well tolerated but can cause transient nausea or other GI disturbances.

Warnings/Precautions

Rule out reversible and potentially treatable causes of dementia before ergoloid mesylate therapy is prescribed. Periodically reevaluate any perceived benefit of therapy to the patient.

Dosing Guidelines

Usual starting dose: 1 mg TID; increase up to 12 mg/d (divided). Results may not be detected for 3 or 4 weeks, and treatment with a minimal dose of 6 mg/d may be needed for at least 6 months to detect any benefit. This product is available in tablet, liquid, and liquid capsule formulations.

CHOLINESTERASE INHIBITORS

Because of the well-documented degeneration of cholinergic neurons in the CNS in AD and the importance of this system in normal memory function, drug development research has focused on agents that restore levels of this neurotransmitter either directly (ie, cholinergic-receptor agonists) or indirectly (ie, cholinesterase inhibitors). Two cholinesterase inhibitors, tacrine (Cognex®; tetrahydroaminoacridine [THA]) (Table 95) and donepezil (Aricept®; Table 98), are approved for the treatment of mild to moderate cognitive impairment of AD. Donepezil, a second-generation agent, is highly specific for brain acetylcholinesterase, whereas tacrine is nonspecific and inhibits peripheral butyrylcholinesterase as well. The specificity of donepezil may have advantages in terms of safety, and possibly efficacy.[194]

TACRINE

Table 95. Overview of tacrine therapy

Feature	Comments
Mechanism	Centrally active, reversible, nonspecific cholinesterase inhibitor, ↑ ACH levels by minimizing or preventing ACH breakdown after release from remaining cholinergic neurons
Pharmacokinetics	Rapid oral absorption, extensive hepatic metabolism via hepatic CYP450 (primarily CYP1A2) (Table 96); liver disease may ↓ elimination. Serum levels ↑ by 50% in females and ↓ by 33% in smokers
Efficacy	Minimal but significant improvement in ADAS cog and global impressions. High rate of withdrawal due to side effects
Safety	GI distress, myalgia, ataxia, anorexia (dose related). ↑ LFTs require extensive and prolonged monitoring
Dosing	10 mg QID (empty stomach, between meals) for ≥6 weeks; ↑ to 20 mg QID if LFTs normal and tolerance good. Discontinue if no response in 6 months

Abbreviations defined in GLOSSARY.

Efficacy

Tacrine does not change the natural, progressive course of AD, and it is relatively ineffective in advanced stages of AD when few cholinergic neurons remain viable. In two key placebo-controlled trials of up to 30 weeks' duration, most patients with mild to moderate probable AD who were taking tacrine (20 to 160 mg/d) showed minimal but statistically significant improvement in the Alzheimer's Disease Assessment Scale cognitive subscale (ADAS cog)[293] and Clinicians' Global Impression measures.[294-296] However, there was a wide range of responses, and a substantial number of patients could not tolerate tacrine therapy and withdrew from the trials. Importantly, the beneficial effects of tacrine tended to diminish with time, even in patients who experienced an initial beneficial response.

Table 96. Common drug and food interactions with tacrine

Interacting substance	Effect of interaction
Anticholinergics	Tacrine may interfere with activity of anticholinergics
Cholinergic agonists (bethanechol), cholinesterase inhibitors (physostigmine), succinylcholine	Tacrine may have a synergistic effect
Theophylline	↓ Elimination of theophylline and ↑ levels. Monitor theophylline levels; ↓ dose accordingly
Cimetidine	Cimetidine ↓ tacrine metabolism: ↑ levels
Food	Food ↓ plasma tacrine levels by one third; take between meals if possible
NSAIDs	May ↑ gastric acid secretion and ↑ risk of GI bleeding

Abbreviations defined in GLOSSARY.

Information in this table obtained from *Physicians' Desk Reference*, *Facts and Comparisons*, or *AHFS Drug Information*. Please refer to those sources for current and additional prescribing information.

Safety

Common adverse events are nausea, vomiting, diarrhea, dyspepsia, other GI symptoms, elevated LFTs (see Warnings/Precautions), myalgia, anorexia, and ataxia. Except for LFT abnormalities and myalgia, these effects are dose related. Do not give tacrine to pregnant or lactating women (Pregnancy Category C; see GLOSSARY; see also DRUG USE IN PREGNANCY/ LACTATION, page 162).

Warnings/Precautions

Use tacrine carefully in patients with current or past liver dysfunction (ie, elevated LFTs). Tacrine commonly increases LFTs in persons without a prior history of liver disease and may cause clinically significant sequelae (eg, jaundice). However, prompt withdrawal of tacrine in such circumstances will only rarely result in liver injury, and LFTs should return to normal limits within 4 to 6 weeks. Patients who develop clinical jaundice (total bilirubin >3 mg/dL) or those with clinical signs or symptoms of hypersensitivity with elevated LFTs should permanently stop tacrine therapy (see Dosing Guidelines, page 154, and prescribing information for LFT monitoring advice).

Tacrine stimulates cholinergic activity and should be used cautiously in selected patients (Table 97).

Table 97. Cautions related to cholinergic activity of tacrine and donepezil

Tacrine may cause	Use with caution in
Bradycardia	"Sick sinus syndrome," conduction abnormalities, bradyarrhythmia
↑ Gastric acid secretion	Patients at risk for ulcers (eg, history of ulcer disease, current NSAID users). Monitor for active or occult GI bleeding
Bladder outflow obstruction	Bladder dysfunction
Seizures	Limited potential; seizures also may be due to AD itself
Asthma	History of asthma

Abbreviations defined in GLOSSARY.

Information in this table obtained from *Physicians' Desk Reference, Facts and Comparisons,* or *AHFS Drug Information.* Please refer to those sources for current and additional prescribing information.

Dosing Guidelines

Prescribe tacrine only when a caregiver can monitor patient compliance with drug administration at regular intervals. Usual starting dose: 10 mg QID; do not increase dose for at least 6 weeks to observe potential delayed LFT elevation. After this time, increase the dose to 20 mg QID if LFTs are normal and patient is tolerating therapy. Give higher doses (eg, 30 to 40 mg QID) at 6-week intervals unless side effects appear. It may take up to 6 months to see any benefit, and if none is seen within this time, discontinue tacrine therapy.

After tacrine therapy is initiated, monitor LFTs every other week for at least the first 16 weeks, monthly for 2 months, and every 3 months subsequently. Reduce the dose by 40 mg/d if LFTs are between three and five times the upper limit of normal. Discontinue tacrine if LFTs are greater than five times the upper limit of normal. If treatment is stopped and restarted for any reason, resume weekly monitoring as described above.

DONEPEZIL

Table 98. Overview of donepezil therapy

Feature	Comments
Mechanism	↑ ACH levels via specific and reversible inhibition of brain cholinesterase
Pharmacokinetics	Nearly complete oral absorption, unaffected by food; peak levels in 4 h. 96% protein bound, extensive metabolism via CYP2D6 and CYP3A4; two active metabolites. QD dosing ($t_{1/2}$ 70 h). Clearance ↓ 20% in cirrhosis[297]
Efficacy	Dose-dependent improvement on ADAS cog and Clinicians' Global Impression scales. Gradual ↓ of clinical benefit upon discontinuation
Safety	Better tolerated than tacrine, especially LFTs. Nausea, diarrhea, vomiting common but cause few treatment discontinuations
Dosing	5 mg HS; ↑ to 10 mg HS after 4 - 6 weeks if needed but unlikely to provide ↑ improvement

Abbreviations defined in GLOSSARY.

Drug Interactions

No significant interactions with theophylline, warfarin, digoxin, cimetidine, or furosemide have been observed (Table 99). Agents that induce CYP2D6 or CYP3A4 could increase donepezil metabolism and reduce its therapeutic effect.

Efficacy

Like tacrine, donepezil has no effect on the natural underlying course of dementia, and its clinical effects may lessen as the disease progresses and fewer cholinergic neurons remain viable. In placebo-controlled studies of up to 30 weeks' duration, patients receiving doses of 1, 3, 5, or 10 mg/d of donepezil showed significant dose-dependent improvement on the ADAS cog (see GLOSSARY) and Clinicians' Global Impression scales.[298-300] Discontinuation of donepezil resulted in a gradual loss of clinical benefit, suggesting that the underlying course of AD is not altered.

Safety

Donepezil is better tolerated than tacrine, especially with regard to effects on LFTs. Common dose-related side effects include nausea, diarrhea, and vomiting; these occurred in 5% to 11% of patients in clinical trials and caused 1% to 3% of patients to discontinue treatment. Syncope was observed (2%). Safety data in lactating and pregnant women (Pregnancy Category C; see

GLOSSARY) are lacking and donepezil should not be used in these patients (see also DRUG USE IN PREGNANCY/LACTATION, page 162).

Table 99. Common drug interactions with donepezil

Interacting drug	Effect of interaction
Anticholinergics	Donepezil may interfere with activity of anticholinergics
Cholinergic agonists (bethanechol), cholinesterase inhibitors (physostigmine), succinylcholine	Donepezil may have a synergistic effect with these drugs
Ketoconazole, quinidine	May ↓ donepezil metabolism; clinical impact unknown
NSAIDs	May ↑ gastric acid secretion; ↑ risk of GI bleeding

Abbreviations defined in GLOSSARY.
Information in this table obtained from *Physicians' Desk Reference, Facts and Comparisons,* or *AHFS Drug Information.* Please refer to those sources for current and additional prescribing information.

Warnings/Precautions
Like tacrine, donepezil stimulates cholinergic activity and should be used cautiously in selected patients (see Table 97).

Dosing Guidelines
Usual starting dose: 5 mg HS; after 4 to 6 weeks, some patients may gain additional benefit from an increase to 10 mg HS.

CHOLINERGIC AGONISTS
Although theoretically appealing, no commercially available drugs of this class have provided clinical utility in patients with AD. Although patients with AD taking bethanechol have shown some improvement on the Mini-Mental State Examination (MMSE), the drug must be given intracerebroventricularly because it does not cross the blood-brain barrier. Other oral agents (eg, pilocarpine) have been ineffective or have required frequent intravenous administration (eg, arecoline). A number of newer orally active cholinergic-receptor agonists are under study.[184]

MISCELLANEOUS
Selegiline (Eldepryl®; formerly L-deprenyl) is used in Parkinson's disease for symptomatic improvement and neuroprotection. The drug also has been effective in improving cognitive function and disturbed behavior (eg, anxiety, cooperation, agitation) in patients with AD[184,301] (Table 100).

Table 100. Overview of selegiline therapy

Feature	Comments
Mechanism	Irreversible, selective inhibition of MAO-B at low doses (≤10 mg/d); selectivity lost at higher doses (eg, ≥20 mg/d). May ↑ dopaminergic activity by other unknown mechanisms; may ↓ progression of AD by reducing oxidative neuronal stress[184]
Pharmacokinetics	Orally absorbed (↑ bioavailability when taken with food), extensive hepatic metabolism; one active metabolite. No data on effects of renal or hepatic impairment
Efficacy	↑ Cognition and behavior
Safety	Nausea, dizziness, abdominal pain, confusion, hallucinations, headache, dry mouth, dyskinesia
Dosing	5 mg BID maximum. Higher doses ↑ side effects and do not improve efficacy

Abbreviations defined in GLOSSARY.

Efficacy

In randomized, placebo-controlled trials, selegiline (10 mg/d) imparts limited improvement of cognition and behavior in patients with AD.[302,303] Lower daily doses may be sufficient for neuroprotection but additional trials are needed.

Safety

Safety data from controlled clinical trials are limited, but nausea, dizziness, abdominal pain, confusion, hallucinations, dry mouth, vivid dreams, dyskinesia, and headache have occurred. Selegiline is rated Pregnancy Category C (see GLOSSARY; see also DRUG USE IN PREGNANCY/LACTATION, page 162).

Warnings/Precautions/Drug Interactions

Do not increase the dose of selegiline to more than 10 mg/d. CNS toxicity (including hyperpyrexia, severe agitation, hallucinations, and death) has occurred in some patients taking selegiline with TCAs, SSRIs, or meperidine. Hypertensive crises have occurred in patients taking selegiline and the sympathomimetic agent ephedrine.

Dosing Guidelines

Usual dose: 5 mg BID (with breakfast and lunch). Higher doses are not more effective and cause more side effects. In trials of AD patients, clinical benefit was evident within a few weeks.

Stimulants

Stimulants used in psychiatry include dextroamphetamine (Dexedrine®), methylphenidate (Ritalin®), and pemoline (Cylert®). These drugs are indicated for the treatment of narcolepsy (ie, daily, irresistible, involuntary sleep attacks) and attention-deficit/hyperactivity disorder (ADHD) in children. Stimulants also have been used to manage obesity, but they are of questionable value.[304] Stimulants can be used in patients with treatment-resistant or -refractory depression and medically ill patients (eg, cancer, stroke, AIDS) with depression in whom typical antidepressants may cause clinically unacceptable side effects. Because these situations are not commonly managed in the primary care setting and because of important abuse and dependence issues, interested readers should refer to reference 304 for further information about the use of stimulants in psychiatry.

Overview of Pharmacotherapy in Primary Care

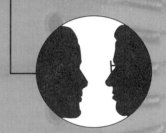

General Principles

The clinical response to psychotropic drugs is individual and based on the severity and duration of the psychiatric disorder, pharmacokinetic features of the drug, and patient factors such as hepatic metabolic capacity, renal function, nutritional status, body weight, presence of concurrent medical conditions, concomitant drug therapy, and others. Nearly all psychotropic drugs can be measured in blood (serum or plasma) but not all need to be. Therapeutic ranges have been established for some psychotropic drugs that may assist in the evaluation of nonresponse, toxicity, or noncompliance. Apparent treatment nonresponse may be related to several factors, such as incorrect diagnosis or inadequate dose or duration of therapy.

In general, the information and guidelines contained in this handbook pertain to otherwise normal, healthy adults. However, there are certain individuals in whom special care is needed when selecting, initiating, and monitoring therapy for mental disorders: the elderly, and pregnant or lactating women.

Drug Use in Pregnancy/Lactation

The high incidence of mental illness in pregnant women and the growing popularity of breast feeding means that clinicians likely will be faced with decisions about the use of psychotropic drugs in pregnant or lactating women or in women wishing to conceive. All of these drugs cross the placenta, but data are limited about potential teratogenic effects, neonatal toxicity, or postnatal behavioral problems (Table 101).[305-308]

No drug is approved for use during pregnancy or lactation. However, the FDA has developed a conservative rating system (see GLOSSARY) that, although by no means definitive, may assist clinicians in choosing therapy during pregnancy. The American Academy of Pediatrics[311] offers a rating system for drugs being considered for use in lactating women. This group considers most antidepressants, antipsychotics, and benzodiazepines as drugs "whose effect on nursing infants is unknown but may be of concern" and lithium as "contraindicated."

GENERAL TREATMENT PRINCIPLES DURING PREGNANCY OR LACTATION

If possible, drug use during the first trimester should be avoided and every attempt made to use nonpharmacologic methods for symptom control during this time. It may be less important to resolve the disorder during the pregnancy rather than simply control symptoms to maintain functional capacity. However, some patients will require pharmacologic treatment because in some cases (eg, psychosis, suicidality), the disorder itself or the reduced functional capacity it causes (eg, maternal malnutrition) may be more detrimental to fetal outcome than the drug itself.[305] Fully disclose the risks and benefits of treatment and nontreatment (eg, relapse) to the patient and family, and the possible risks of infant drug exposure. If a depressed woman wishes to conceive yet remain on antidepressant therapy during this time, an agent such as a short-acting SSRI (eg, paroxetine, fluvoxamine, sertraline) may be preferred because it can be easily discontinued after documentation of pregnancy, prior to the establishment of fetoplacental circulation.[305] If drug therapy is needed in a pregnant woman, use the lowest effective dose for the shortest time necessary to minimize in utero exposure as well as infant exposure during breast feeding. Physiologic changes during pregnancy (eg, delayed gastric emptying and GI motility, increased body fat and total body water, decreased protein binding, and increased metabolism) may necessitate use of higher doses as compared with those used prior to pregnancy. The recommendations in Table 102 are provided for guidance only; consult additional resources whenever possible.

Table 101. Risks associated with psychotropic drugs during pregnancy and lactation[233,305,306,308-310]

Drug class	Possible risks
TCA	No clear association with fetal malformations; fetal withdrawal syndrome, tachycardia, GI obstruction (anticholinergic effects) reported. Secondary amines (see Table 41) generally recommended. Most TCAs found in low amounts in breast milk; doxepin not recommended during lactation (high milk/plasma ratio[a])
MAOI	Fetal malformations (tranylcypromine). Rarely used during pregnancy because of dietary restrictions and side effects
SSRI	Growing database shows no apparent fetal anomalies. Milk/plasma ratios[a]: citalopram (3) > sertraline (2.3) > fluoxetine (0.29 - 1.51) > fluvoxamine (0.29) > paroxetine (0.09)
Miscellaneous antidepressants in breast milk	Very limited data (isolated case reports). Bupropion found in low quantities
Antipsychotics	Large database (pregnancy-related emesis). Small but ↑ risk of some congenital malformations, perinatal syndrome (restlessness, tremor); ↓ risk after 1st trimester; piperazine or piperidine[b] agents may be less teratogenic
Drugs for EPS	Orofacial clefts, withdrawal syndrome (diphenhydramine); adverse effects on fetal GI motility/obstruction (anticholinergics); animal teratogen (amantadine)
Benzodiazepines	Orofacial cleft (highly controversial); fetal withdrawal syndrome
Lithium	Congenital cardiovascular malformations (Ebstein's anomaly), neonatal lithium toxicity (floppy baby, cyanosis); avoid during lactation (↑ potential for toxicity linked to poor infant hydration)
Mood-stabilizing anticonvulsants[c]	Spina bifida, intrauterine growth retardation, orofacial cleft. Compatible with breast feeding

Abbreviations defined in GLOSSARY.

[a]A lower milk/plasma ratio indicates less infant exposure to the drug.

[b]See Table 80.

[c]Data from observations in epileptic women; limited data in women with bipolar disorder.

Table 102. Treatment recommendations for some psychiatric disorders during pregnancy[305]

Disorder	Recommendations
Schizophrenia	Mild, new-onset psychosis: PRN antipsychotic use; chronic psychosis, frequent relapse: maintain usual regimen
Major depression	New-onset or mild/moderate symptoms: nondrug approaches during 1st trimester; use SSRIs or secondary amine TCAs (see Table 41). Avoid MAOIs. Hospitalize for severe symptoms; consider ECT
Bipolar disorder	Slowly taper lithium before conception, if possible. If used during pregnancy, higher doses may be needed but taper by 30% at the onset of labor to ↓ maternal and neonatal toxicity caused by fluid shifts. Hospitalize for severe psychosis. If prior nonresponse to lithium, give folic acid (4 mg QD) with anticonvulsant mood stabilizer (eg, divalproex sodium) before conception and during 1st trimester. Prescribe vitamin K before delivery to improve clotting ability
PD	Taper prior to conception if possible; use nondrug measures. Use SSRIs, TCAs, and benzodiazepines if absolutely necessary
OCD	Use nondrug approaches first; SSRI preferred. Clomipramine acceptable but ↑ orthostatic hypotension; also neonatal seizures during labor and delivery
Eating disorders	Nondrug approaches with TCAs or SSRIs

Abbreviations defined in GLOSSARY.

Drug Use in the Elderly

Typically, elderly patients (ie, >65 years of age) make up a substantial proportion (possibly 40% or more) of a primary care physician's patient base,[312] and with the aging of America, this trend is not likely to reverse itself.

The use of psychoactive drugs in elderly patients differs somewhat from that in younger adults because of physiologic changes associated with aging, the presence of concurrent diseases, and a greater risk of drug toxicity and drug interactions related to polypharmacy (Table 103).

Table 103. Factors affecting use of psychopharmacologic drugs in the elderly[312,313]

Factor	Examples and implications
• Age-related physiologic changes: – body composition (altered fat:muscle ratio)	↑ Distribution and prolonged clearance of fat-soluble drugs causes ↑ therapeutic and toxic effects
– CNS structure or function	↑ Sensitivity to therapeutic and toxic CNS effects of drugs
– ↓ renal or hepatic function	↓ Metabolism or elimination may ↑ blood levels
• ↑ Susceptibility to ADRs	↑ Direct toxicity (eg, anticholinergic effects, sedation, EPS)
	↑ Indirect toxicity (eg, falls, accidents caused by ↑ sedation)
• Chronic medical problems (eg, malnutrition, liver disease)	>80% of elderly Americans have ≥1 chronic medical problem. May ↑ blood levels of some drugs (↓ protein binding, ↓ metabolism)
• Polypharmacy	Elderly Americans receive one third of all prescriptions. ↑ Risk of drug interactions
• Functional disability	↓ Compliance with regimen if unable to self-medicate or if patient cannot keep scheduled appointments because of lack of reliable transportation
• Cost issues	Elderly on fixed incomes may not fill expensive prescriptions; lack of insurance coverage for drug monitoring or laboratory tests

Abbreviations defined in GLOSSARY.

GENERAL TREATMENT PRINCIPLES IN THE ELDERLY

Before prescribing psychopharmacologic drugs for a presumed mental disorder, rule out and treat possible medical causes of psychiatric presentations. For example, insomnia may be caused by nocturnal angina, gastroesophageal reflux, or leg pain. Agitation or psychosis may be caused by drug toxicity, loneliness, frustration, or pain. Whenever possible, encourage use of nonpharmacologic measures (eg, sleep hygiene measures for insomnia). Remember that the elderly are especially sensitive to both therapeutic and toxic drug effects at any given dose or blood level. The adage "start low and go slow" is important in this population; for many drugs, one third to one half the usual adult dose will provide the desired therapeutic effect. Finally, because the elderly are more sensitive to side effects of psychopharmacologic drugs, base treatment selection on not only efficacy but also side-effect profiles (Table 104).

Table 104. Treatment recommendations for some psychiatric disorders in the elderly[312,313]

Disorder	Generally prefer	Generally avoid
Anxiety	Benzodiazepines, buspirone	Antidepressants, antihistamines, barbiturates
Depression	SSRIs, secondary amine TCAs,[a] trazodone, bupropion	MAOIs (unless treating atypical depression)
Insomnia	Benzodiazepines, zolpidem	Antidepressants, antihistamines (including OTC), barbiturates, nonbarbiturate hypnotics
Mania	Lithium, valproic acid	—
Psychosis, agitation	Antipsychotics,[b] trazodone, anticonvulsants	Antihistamines, barbiturates, benzodiazepines, SSRIs

Abbreviations defined in GLOSSARY.
[a]See Table 41.
[b]See Table 82.

Resources

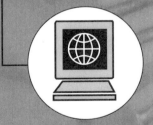

GENERAL MENTAL HEALTH ORGANIZATIONS

American Psychiatric Association (APA)
1400 K Street, NW
Washington, DC 20005
TEL: 202-282-6000
Web site: http://www.psych.org; e-mail: apa@psych.org

This national medical specialty society publishes the Diagnostic and Statistical Manual of Mental Disorders, 4th edition, Primary Care Version *and an informative patient information pamphlet series called* "Let's Talk Facts About Mental Illness."

National Alliance for the Mentally Ill (NAMI)
200 North Glebe Road, Suite 1015
Arlington, VA 22201
TEL: 703-524-7600 or 1-800-950-NAMI (1-800-950-6264)
(24-hour message line available 7 days a week)
Web site: http://www.nami.org; e-mail: namioffc@aol.com

A nonprofit, self-help support and advocacy organization for consumers, friends, and families of people with severe mental illness. Provides written materials on mental illness.

National Institute of Mental Health (NIMH)
Office of Scientific Information
5600 Fishers Lane
Room 7-99
Rockville, MD 20892-8032
TEL: 301-443-4536
Web site: http://www.nimh.nih.gov; e-mail: nimhinfo@nih.gov

Conducts and supports research nationwide on mental illness and mental health. Part of National Institutes of Health (NIH), which is a component of the US Department of Health and Human Services.

National Mental Health Association (NMHA)
1021 Prince Street
Alexandria, VA 22314-2971
TEL: 703-684-7722 or 1-800-969-NMHA (1-800-969-6642) (information center)
Web site: http://www.nmha.org; e-mail: nmhainfo@aol.com

Nonprofit mental health advocacy group providing free pamphlets and fact sheets on more than 200 mental health topics, referral to local mental health care providers, and a directory of networks of local mental health care associations.

ALZHEIMER'S DISEASE

http://www.Alzheimers.com
A physician-authored gateway to information about Alzheimer's disease on the Internet.

Alzheimer's Disease and Related Disorders Association (ADRDA),
also known as **Alzheimer's Association (AA)**
919 North Michigan Avenue
Suite 1000
Chicago, IL 60611-1676
TEL: 312-335-8700 or 1-800-272-3900; (24-hour hotline: 1-800-621-0379)
Web site: http://www.alz.org; e-mail: INFO@alz.org

National nonprofit organization with extensive family-oriented information and newsletter. Local chapters are an excellent resource for information on community services (eg, adult day care, respite programs).

Alzheimer's Disease Centers (ADC)
Offers diagnosis and management services (costs are variable), information about AD and local resources, opportunities to participate in drug trials. Contact ADEAR (below) for nearest center.

Alzheimer's Disease Education and Referral Program (ADEAR)
ADEAR Center
Box 8250
Silver Spring, MD 20907-8250
TEL: 1-800-438-4380 or 301-495-3311

Sponsored by the National Institute on Aging, this is a national clearinghouse for information on AD. ADEAR performs free literature searches on AD for clinicians and researchers. Also offers information and publications on diagnosis, treatment, care giving, and long-term care issues.

American Association of Retired Persons (AARP)
601 E Street, NW
Washington, DC 20049
TEL: 1-800-424-3410
Web site: http://www.aarp.org; e-mail: member@aarp.org

A nonprofit, nonpartisan organization dedicated to helping older Americans achieve lives of dignity and purpose. Provides literature on services and legislative issues for older adults. Numerous state and regional offices listed in telephone book.

Area Agency on Aging
Division of the US Department of Health and Human Services; coordinates a large network of offices on aging to provide information and referrals. Check local listing for nearest Area Agency on Aging.

Eldercare Locator
927 15th Street, NW
6th Floor
Washington, DC 20005
TEL: 1-800-677-1116

A service of the Administration on Aging, US Department of Health and Human Services, and is administered by the National Association of Area Agencies on Aging. Provides information and referrals to respite care and community care agencies.

ANXIETY DISORDERS

Anxiety Disorders Association of America (ADAA)
11900 Parklawn Drive
Suite 100
Rockville, MD 20852-2624
TEL: 301-231-9350
Web site: http://www.adaa.org

Promotes prevention and cure of anxiety disorders.

OCD Foundation, Inc (Obsessive-Compulsive Disorder)
PO Box 70
Milford, CT 06460
TEL: 203-878-5669

DEPRESSION/MOOD DISORDERS

Agency for Health Care Policy and Research (AHCPR)
Executive Office Center
2101 East Jefferson Street
Suite 401
Rockville, MD 20852

Publishes "Clinical Practice Guideline: Depression in Primary Care."
To order, call or write AHCPR Publications Clearinghouse, PO Box 8547, Silver Spring, MD 20907; TEL: 1-800-358-9295.

American Foundation for Suicide Prevention (AFSP)
120 Wall Street
22nd Floor
New York, NY 10005
TEL: 888-333-AFSP (888-333-2377) or 212-363-3500
Web site: http://www.afsp.org

Depression/Awareness, Recognition and Treatment (D/ART)
(affiliated with NIMH; TEL: 301-443-4536)

Provides outreach programs for patients, consumers, health professionals, focuses on increasing public awareness, and encourages recognition and treatment of depression. Print materials and other programs available.

National Alliance for Research on Schizophrenia and Depression (NARSAD)
60 Cutter Mill Road
Suite 404
Great Neck, NY 11021
TEL: 516-829-0091
Web site: http://www.mhsource.com

National, nonprofit provider of funds for mental illness research.

National Depressive and Manic Depressive Association (NDMDA)
730 North Franklin
Suite 501
Chicago, IL 60610
TEL: 312-642-0049 or 1-800-82-NDMDA (1-800-826-3632)
Web site: http://www.ndmda.org

Largest patient advocacy group in the United States. Provides information on bipolar disorder and depression for affected individuals, family members, the public, and the media.

National Foundation for Depressive Illness, Inc
PO Box 2257
New York, NY 10116
TEL: 1-800-248-4344

Nonprofit organization offering a recorded patient hotline about symptoms of depression, manic-depressive illness, and a printed bibliography.

SCHIZOPHRENIA

http://www.schizophrenia.com
Link to resources about schizophrenia on the Internet.

Recovery, Incorporated
Self-help group similar to Alcoholics Anonymous.

National Alliance for Research on Schizophrenia and Depression (NARSAD)
60 Cutter Mill Road
Suite 404
Great Neck, NY 11021
TEL: 516-829-0091
Web site: http://www.mhsource.com

National, nonprofit provider of funds for mental illness research.

SLEEP DISORDERS

American Sleep Disorders Association (ASDA)
1610 14th Street, NW
Suite 300
Rochester, MN 55901-2200
TEL: 507-287-6006
Web site: http://www.asda.org; e-mail: asda@asda.org

Provides professional and patient information on sleep medicine and sleep research.

National Sleep Foundation (NSF)

729 15th Street, NW
4th Floor
Washington, DC 20005
Web site: http://www.sleepfoundation.org; e-mail: natsleep@erols.com

A nonprofit organization promoting public understanding of sleep and sleep disorders. Supports sleep-related education, research, and advocacy to improve public health and safety.

SUBSTANCE ABUSE DISORDERS

National Institute on Drug Abuse (NIDA)

Web site: http://www.nida.nih.gov; e-mail: information@lists.nida.nih.gov

Check local telephone directories for 24-hour helpline and assistance services for alcohol, cocaine, and narcotics abuse. Also listed are local or state-wide listings for:

Alcoholics Anonymous

Web site: http://www.alcoholics-anonymous.org

Cocaine Anonymous

Web site: http://www.ca.org

Marijuana Anonymous

Narcotics Anonymous

Web site: http://www.na.org

PUBLICATIONS

To order *"Clinical Practice Guideline: Depression in Primary Care"* or *"Clinical Practice Guideline: Smoking Cessation,"* call or write AHCPR Publications Clearinghouse, PO Box 8547, Silver Spring, MD 20907; TEL: 1-800-358-9295.

The National Guideline Clearinghouse also can be accessed on the Internet: http://www.guideline.gov. This site contains several hundred clinical practice guidelines and can be searched by disease or condition, by treatment or intervention, or by the name of the submitting organization.

Glossary/Bibliography/
Appendices/Index

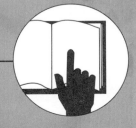

Glossary

ACH: acetylcholine

AD: Alzheimer's disease

ADAS cog: Alzheimer's Disease Assessment Scale, cognitive subscale. This scale examines memory attention, reason, language, and praxis

ADHD: attention-deficit/hyperactivity disorder

ADR: adverse drug reaction

AHCPR: Agency for Health Care Policy and Research

AIDS: acquired immunodeficiency syndrome

AN: anorexia nervosa

BID: twice daily

BN: bulimia nervosa

BP: blood pressure

BPH: benign prostatic hyperplasia

BUN: blood urea nitrogen

CAD: coronary artery disease

CBC: complete blood count

CBT: cognitive-behavioral therapy

CCK: cholecystokinin

ChAT: choline acetyltransferase

CHF: congestive heart failure

CNS: central nervous system

Comorbidity: presence of two or more psychiatric disorders existing simultaneously. Especially common with depressive and anxiety disorders

CrCl: creatinine clearance

CRF: corticotropin-releasing factor

CSF: cerebrospinal fluid

CT: computed tomography

Cytochrome P450 system (CYP450): proteins that catalyze oxidative drug metabolism. Many families and subfamilies of isoenzymes. Cytochromes (CYP) 1A2, 2C, 2D6, and 3A4 are relevant to metabolism of many psychotherapeutic agents and clinically important drug interactions (see reference 213 for review)

DA: dopamine

DEA: Drug Enforcement Agency

Delusions: erroneous beliefs involving misinterpretation of perceptions or experiences (eg, belief that one is being tormented or followed). Bizarre delusions are implausible, not understandable, and not related to typical life experiences (eg, belief that one's internal organs have been removed and replaced or that aliens have inserted thoughts into one's mind)[13]

DSM-IV: *Diagnostic and Statistical Manual of Mental Disorders*, fourth edition

DST: dexamethasone suppression test

ECG: electrocardiogram

ECT: electroconvulsive therapy

EEG: electroencephalogram

EPS: extrapyramidal side effects; common with antipsychotic therapy and are due to a relative imbalance between dopaminergic and cholinergic function. Includes *acute dystonic reactions* (eg, facial grimacing, oculogyric crisis), *akathisia* (ie, subjective feeling of restlessness and objective restless movement), *pseudoparkinson* features (eg, slowed movement, masked facies, rigidity, resting tremor) and *tardive dyskinesia* (ie, irregular facial movements). Drug-induced EPS are managed by lowering the antipsychotic drug dose or with anticholinergic, antihistaminergic, or dopaminergic agents

ESR: erythrocyte sedimentation rate

FDA: United States Food and Drug Administration

FLY-BOCS: Florida Yale-Brown Obsessive Compulsive Scale

GABA: γ-aminobutyric acid, an inhibitory neurotransmitter

GAD: generalized anxiety disorder

GGT: γ-glutamyltransferase

GH: growth hormone

GI: gastrointestinal

Hallucinations: sensory misperceptions (eg, auditory, visual, olfactory, tactile, gustatory). In schizophrenia, auditory hallucinations are the most common

HAM-D: Hamilton Rating Scale for Depression

HIV: human immunodeficiency virus

HPA: hypothalamic-pituitary-adrenal axis

HPT: hypothalamic-pituitary-thyroid axis

HS: bedtime

5-HT: 5-hydroxytryptamine, serotonin

IM: intramuscular

IV: intravenous

LFTs: liver function tests such as alanine aminotransferase (ALT [formerly SGPT]), aspartate aminotransferase (AST [formerly SGOT]), γ-glutamyltransferase (GGT), bilirubin

MADRS: Montgomery Asberg Depression Rating Scale

MAOI: monoamine oxidase inhibitor. Monoamine oxidase is responsible for the breakdown of dopamine, serotonin, and norepinephrine. Two types: MAO-A and MAO-B (found primarily in the brain)

MCV: mean corpuscular volume

MI: myocardial infarction

MINI: Mini International Neuropsychiatric Interview

MMSE: Mini Mental State Examination: a short (<10 minutes to administer), structured (11 questions) clinician-administered examination of cognitive aspects of mental function.[189] Good for initial and serial measurement of mental function; reliable over time

MRI: magnetic resonance imaging

NE: norepinephrine

Neuritic plaques: also called senile plaques. Like NFT, a hallmark neurohistologic feature of AD. Neuritic plaques have a central core of insoluble ß-amyloid protein surrounded by distended and abnormal dendrites and small axons

NFT: neurofibrillary tangles. A neurohistologic feature of AD consisting of filament bundles in cell bodies, axons, and dendrites found in the cerebral cortex and hippocampus. NFT density closely correlated with degree of cognitive impairment

NMS: neuroleptic malignant syndrome; a rare, idiosyncratic complication of antipsychotic therapy that includes EPS (mainly muscle rigidity), hyperthermia, autonomic instability (ie, tachycardia, hypertension, dysrhythmia), and varying degrees of consciousness. Potentially fatal respiratory failure can occur. Treatment involves discontinuation of the antipsychotic, and intensive symptomatic treatment. NMS may recur if antipsychotic therapy is restarted

NSAID: nonsteroidal anti-inflammatory drug (eg, ibuprofen, indomethacin, naproxen, etc)

OCD: obsessive-compulsive disorder

OTC: over-the-counter (nonprescription) medications

PD: panic disorder

PET: positron emission tomography

Pregnancy Categories: The FDA has established five categories for classifying drugs for use during pregnancy

Category A: Adequate well-controlled studies in pregnant women have not demonstrated fetal risk in the first trimester and no evidence of risk in later trimesters

Category B: No fetal risk in animal studies but no adequate studies in pregnant women. Or, animal studies have shown adverse effect but adequate studies in pregnant women have not demonstrated fetal risk during the first trimester and no evidence of risk in later trimesters

Category C: No adverse effect in animal studies but no adequate studies in humans. Benefits from use of the drug by pregnant women may be acceptable despite these risks. Or, no animal reproduction studies and no adequate human studies

Category D: Evidence of human fetal risk but potential benefits in pregnant women may be acceptable despite these risks

Category X: Animal or human studies demonstrate fetal abnormalities or evidence of fetal risk; risk of use clearly outweighs any possible benefit (contraindicated)

PRN: as needed

PT: prothrombin time

PTSD: posttraumatic stress disorder

QD: once daily

QID: four times daily

QOD: every other day

REM: rapid eye movement

Serotonin syndrome: a syndrome resembling NMS and consisting of abdominal pain, sweating, myoclonus, delirium, ↑ BP, seizures, fever, tachycardia, and possibly coma

SIADH: syndrome of inappropriate antidiuretic hormone

SPECT: single positron emission computed tomography

SSRI: selective serotonin reuptake inhibitor. Class of antidepressants includes fluoxetine, paroxetine, sertraline, citalopram, and fluvoxamine (currently not indicated for the treatment of depression)

$t_{1/2}$: elimination half-life

Tardive dyskinesia (TD): syndrome of potentially irreversible, involuntary dyskinetic movements. Unpredictable, but more likely in elderly women. Risk increases with duration of antipsychotic treatment and total cumulative dose. No known treatment except withdrawal of the antipsychotic

TCA: tricyclic antidepressant

TFTs: thyroid function tests

TID: three times daily

T_{max}: time to reach maximum plasma or serum concentration

TOP-8 Scale: Treatment Outcome PTSD Scale

TRH: thyrotropin-releasing hormone

TSH: thyroid-stimulating hormone

WBC: white blood cell

Bibliography

1.   Higgins ES. A review of unrecognized mental illness in primary care: prevalence, natural history, and efforts to change the course. *Arch Fam Med*. 1994;3:908-917.

2.   Sartorius N. Psychiatry in the framework of primary health care: a threat or boost to psychiatry? *Am J Psychiatry*. 1997;154(June suppl): 67-72.

3.   Kessler RC, McGonagle KA, Zhao S, et al. Lifetime and 12-month prevalence of DSM-III-R psychiatric disorders in the United States: results from the National Comorbidity Survey. *Arch Gen Psychiatry*. 1994;51:8-19.

4.   Regier DA, Goldberg ID, Taube CA. The de facto US mental health services system: a public health perspective. *Arch Gen Psychiatry*. 1978;35:685-693.

5.   Schurman RA, Kramer PD, Mitchell JB. The hidden mental health network: treatment of mental illness by nonpsychiatrist physicians. *Arch Gen Psychiatry*. 1985;42:89-94.

6.   Sheikh JI. Anxiety disorders and their treatment. *Clin Geriatr Med*. 1992;8:411-426.

7.   Sherbourne CD, Jackson CA, Meredith LS, Camp P, Wells KB. Prevalence of comorbid anxiety disorders in primary care outpatients. *Arch Fam Med*. 1996;5:27-34.

8.   Katon W, Vitaliano PP, Russo J, Cormier L, Anderson K, Jones M. Panic disorder: epidemiology in primary care. *J Fam Pract*. 1986;23:233-239.

9.   Weissman MM, Bland RC, Canino GJ, et al. The cross-national epidemiology of panic disorder. *Arch Gen Psychiatry*. 1997;54:305-309.

10.   Eaton WW, Kessler RC, Wittchen HU, Magee WJ. Panic and panic disorder in the United States. *Am J Psychiatry*. 1994;151:413-420.

11.   Hirschfeld RMA. Panic disorder: diagnosis, epidemiology, and clinical course. *J Clin Psychiatry*. 1996;57(suppl 10):3-8.

12.   American Psychiatric Association. Practice guideline for the treatment of patients with panic disorder. *Am J Psychiatry*. 1998;155(May suppl):1-34.

13.   American Psychiatric Association. *Diagnostic and Statistical Manual of Mental Disorders*. 4th ed. Washington, DC: American Psychiatric Association; 1994.

14.   Gorman JM, Coplan JD. Comorbidity of depression and panic disorder. *J Clin Psychiatry*. 1996;57(suppl 10):34-41.

15.   Johnson MR, Lydiard RB, Ballenger JC. Panic disorder: pathophysiology and treatment. *Drugs*. 1995;49:328-344.

16. Krystal JH, Deutsch DN, Charney DS. The biological basis of panic disorder. *J Clin Psychiatry.* 1996;57(suppl 10):23-31.

17. Taylor CB. Treatment of anxiety disorders. In: Schatzberg AF, Nemeroff CB, eds. *Textbook of Psychopharmacology.* 2nd ed. Washington, DC: American Psychiatric Press Inc; 1998:775-789.

18. Katon W. Panic disorder: relationship to high medical utilization, unexplained physical symptoms, and medical costs. *J Clin Psychiatry.* 1996;47(suppl 10):11-18.

19. Shear MK. Psychotherapy for panic disorder. *Psychiatr Q.* 1995; 66:321-328.

20. Coplan JD, Pine DS, Papp LA, Gorman JM. An algorithm-oriented treatment approach for panic disorder. *Psychiatric Ann.* 1996;26:192-201.

21. Elliott RL. Panic disorder in primary care. *Prim Psychiatry.* 1995; (September):52-59.

22. Ballenger JC, Wheadon DE, Steiner M, Bushnell W, Gergel IP. Double-blind, fixed-dose, placebo-controlled study of paroxetine in the treatment of panic disorder. *Am J Psychiatry.* 1998;155:36-42.

23. Black DW, Wesner R, Bowers W, Gabel J. A comparison of fluvoxamine, cognitive therapy, and placebo in the treatment of panic disorder. *Arch Gen Psychiatry.* 1993;50:44-50.

24. Boyer W. Serotonin uptake inhibitors are superior to imipramine and alprazolam in alleviating panic attacks: a meta-analysis. *Int Clin Psychopharmacol.* 1995;10:45-49.

25. DeVane CL. The place of selective serotonin reuptake inhibitors in the treatment of panic disorder. *Pharmacotherapy.* 1997;17:282-292.

26. Gunasekara NS, Noble S, Benfield P. Paroxetine: an update of its pharmacology and therapeutic use in depression and a review of its use in other disorders. *Drugs.* 1998;55:85-120.

27. Sheehan DV, Harnett-Sheehan K. The role of SSRIs in panic disorder. *J Clin Psychiatry.* 1996;57(suppl 10):51-58.

28. Rasmussen SA, Eisen JL. The epidemiology and differential diagnosis of obsessive-compulsive disorder. *J Clin Psychiatry.* 1994;55(suppl 10): 5-10.

29. Jenike MA. Obsessive-compulsive and related disorders: a hidden epidemic. *N Engl J Med.* 1989;321:539-541.

30. Zetin M, Kramer MA. Obsessive-compulsive disorder. *Hosp Commun Psychiatry.* 1992;43:689-699.

31. Karno M, Golding JM, Sorenson SB, Burnam MA. The epidemiology of obsessive-compulsive disorder in five US communities. *Arch Gen Psychiatry.* 1988;45:1094-1099.

32. Stein MB, Uhde TW. Biology of anxiety disorders. In: Schatzberg AF, Nemeroff CB, eds. *Textbook of Psychopharmacology.* 2nd ed. Washington, DC: American Psychiatric Press Inc; 1998:609-628.

33. Pigott TA. OCD: where the serotonin selectivity story begins. *J Clin Psychiatry.* 1996;57(suppl 6):11-20.

34. Sichel DA, Cohen LS, Dimmock JA, Rosenbaum JF. Postpartum obsessive-compulsive disorder: a case series. *J Clin Psychiatry.* 1993; 54:156-159.

35. Kim SW, Dysken MW, Kuskowski M. The Yale-Brown Obsessive-Compulsive Scale: a reliability and validity study. *Psychiatry Res.* 1990; 34:99-106.

36. Baer L. Behavior therapy for obsessive-compulsive disorder in the office-based practice. *J Clin Psychiatry.* 1993;54(suppl 6):10-15.

37. Goodman WK, McDougle CJ, Barr LC, Aronson SC, Price LH. Biological approaches to treatment-resistant obsessive-compulsive disorder. *J Clin Psychiatry.* 1993;54(suppl 6):16-26.

38. Jefferson JW, Greist JH. The pharmacotherapy of obsessive-compulsive disorder. *Psychiatric Ann.* 1996;26:202-209.

39. March JS, Frances A, Carpenter D, Kahn DA. Treatment of obsessive-compulsive disorder. Expert Consensus Guidelines Series. *J Clin Psychiatry.* 1997;58(suppl 4):3-72.

40. The Clomipramine Collaborative Study Group. Clomipramine in the treatment of patients with obsessive-compulsive disorder. *Arch Gen Psychiatry.* 1991;48:730-738.

41. Katz RJ, DeVeaugh-Geiss J, Landau P. Clomipramine in obsessive-compulsive disorder. *Biol Psychiatry.* 1990;28:401-414.

42. Pigott TA, Pato MT, Bernstein SE, et al. Controlled comparisons of clomipramine and fluoxetine in the treatment of obsessive-compulsive disorder. *Arch Gen Psychiatry.* 1990;47:926-932.

43. Steiner M, Bushnell WP, Gergel I, Wheadon DE. Long-term treatment and prevention of relapse of obsessive-compulsive disorder with paroxetine. Presented at American Psychiatric Association Annual Meeting; May 1995; Miami, FL.

44. Helzer JE, Robins LN, McEvoy L. Posttraumatic stress disorder in the general population: findings of the Epidemiologic Catchment Area Survey. *N Engl J Med.* 1987;317:1630-1634.

45. Kessler RC, Sonnega A, Bromet E, Hughes M, Nelson CB. Post-traumatic stress disorder in the National Comorbidity Survey. *Arch Gen Psychiatry.* 1995;52:1048-1060.

46. Bremner JD, Southwick SM, Darnell A, Charney DS. Chronic PTSD in Vietnam combat veterans: course of illness and substance abuse. *Am J Psychiatry.* 1996;153:369-375.

47. Deering CG, Glover SG, Ready D, Eddleman HC, Alarcon RD. Unique patterns of comorbidity in posttraumatic stress disorder from different sources of trauma. *Compr Psychiatry.* 1996;37:336-346.

48. Marshall RD, Stein DJ, Liebowitz MR, Yehuda R. A pharmacotherapy algorithm in the treatment of posttraumatic stress disorder. *Psychiatr Ann.* 1996;26:217-226.

49. Orsillo SM, Heimberg RG, Huster HR, Garrett J. Social anxiety disorder and PTSD in Vietnam veterans. *J Trauma Stress.* 1996;9:235-252.

50. Charney DS, Deutch AY, Krystal JH, Southwick SM, Davis M. Psycho-biologic mechanisms of posttraumatic stress disorder. *Arch Gen Psychiatry.* 1993;50:294-305.

51. Marmar CR, Schoenfeld F, Weiss DS, et al. Open trial of fluvoxamine treatment for combat-related posttraumatic stress disorder. *J Clin Psychiatry.* 1996;57(suppl 8):66-72.

52. Bremner JD, Licinio J, Darnell A, et al. Elevated CSF corticotropin-releasing factor concentrations in posttraumatic stress disorder. *Am J Psychiatry.* 1997;154:624-629.

53. Gaston L, Brunet A, Koszycki D, Bradwejn J. MMPI profiles of acute and chronic PTSD in a civilian sample. *J Trauma Stress.* 1996;9:817-832.

54. Solomon SD, Gerrity ET, Muff AM. Efficacy of treatments for posttrau-matic stress disorder: an empirical review. *JAMA.* 1992;268:633-638.

55. van der Kolk BA, Dreyfuss D, Michaels M, et al. Fluoxetine in post-traumatic stress disorder. *J Clin Psychiatry.* 1994;55:517-522.

56. Rothbaum BO, Ninan PT, Thomas L. Sertraline in the treatment of rape victims with posttraumatic stress disorder. *J Trauma Stress.* 1996; 9:865-871.

57. Hertzberg MA, Feldman ME, Beckham JC, Davidson JRT. Trial of trazodone for posttraumatic stress disorder using a multiple baseline group design. *J Clin Psychopharmacol.* 1996;16:294-298.

58. Kosten TR, Frank JB, Dan E, McDougle CJ, Giller EL Jr. Pharmacotherapy for posttraumatic stress disorder using phenelzine or imipramine. *J Nerv Ment Dis.* 1991;179:366-370.

59. Ford N. The use of anticonvulsants in posttraumatic stress disorder: case study and overview. *J Trauma Stress.* 1996;9:857-863.

60. Wittchen H-U, Zhao S, Kessler RC, Eaton WW. DSM-III-R generalized anxiety disorder in the National Comorbidity Survey. *Arch Gen Psychiatry.* 1994;51:355-364.

61. Rickels K, Schweizer E. The treatment of generalized anxiety disorder in patients with depressive symptomatology. *J Clin Psychiatry.* 1993; 54(suppl 1):20-23.

62. Brawman-Mintzer O, Lydiard RB. Biological basis of generalized anxiety disorder. *J Clin Psychiatry.* 1997;58(suppl 3):16-25.

63. Mancuso DM, Townsend MH, Mercante DE. Long-term follow-up of generalized anxiety disorder. *Compr Psychiatry.* 1993;34:441-446.

64. Thompson PM. Generalized anxiety disorder treatment algorithm. *Psychiatr Ann.* 1996;26:227-232.

65. Rocca P, Fonzo V, Scotta M, Zaralda E, Ravizza L. Paroxetine efficacy in the treatment of generalized anxiety disorder. *Acta Psychiatr Scand.* 1997;95:444-450.

66. Schweizer E, Rickels K. Strategies for treatment of generalized anxiety disorder in the primary care setting. *J Clin Psychiatry.* 1997;58(suppl 3):27-31.

67. Nunes EV, McGrath PJ, Quitkin FM. Treating anxiety in patients with alcoholism. *J Clin Psychiatry.* 1995;56(suppl 2):3-9.

68. Rickels K, Downing R, Schweizer E, Hassman H. Antidepressants for the treatment of generalized anxiety disorder: a placebo-controlled comparison of imipramine, trazodone, and diazepam. *Arch Gen Psychiatry.* 1993;50:884-895.

69. Hoehn-Saric R, McLeod DR, Zimmerli WD. Differential effects of alprazolam and imipramine in generalized anxiety disorder: somatic versus psychic symptoms. *J Clin Psychiatry.* 1988;49:293-301.

70. Gammans RE, Stringfellow JC, Hvizdos AJ, et al. Use of buspirone in patients with generalized anxiety disorder and coexisting depressive symptoms. *Pharmacopsychiatry.* 1992;25:193-201.

71. Marshall RD, Schneier FR. An algorithm for the pharmacotherapy of social anxiety disorder. *Psychiatric Ann.* 1996;26:210-216.

72. Davidson JRT, Hughes DC, George LK, Blazer DG. The boundary of social anxiety disorder: exploring the threshold. *Arch Gen Psychiatry.* 1994;51:975-983.

73. Weiller E, Bisserbe J-C, Boyer P, Lepine J-P, Lecrubier Y. Social anxiety disorder in general health care: an unrecognized, undertreated, disabling disorder. *Br J Psychiatry.* 1996;168:169-174.

74. Kessler RC, Stein MB, Berglund P. Social anxiety disorder subtypes in the National Comorbidity Survey. *Am J Psychiatry*. 1998;155:613-619.

75. Hirschfeld RMA. The impact of health care reform on social anxiety disorder. *J Clin Psychiatry*. 1995;56(suppl 5):13-17.

76. Fyer AJ. Heritability of social anxiety: a brief review. *J Clin Psychiatry*. 1993;54(suppl 12):10-12.

77. Davidson JRT, Krishnan KRR, Charles HC, et al. Magnetic resonance spectroscopy in social anxiety disorder: preliminary findings. *J Clin Psychiatry*. 1993;54(suppl 12):19-25.

78. Schneier FR, Johnson J, Hornig CD, et al. Social anxiety disorder: comorbidity and morbidity in an epidemiologic sample. *Arch Gen Psychiatry*. 1992;49:282-288.

79. Greist JH. The diagnosis of social anxiety disorder. *J Clin Psychiatry*. 1995;56(suppl 5):5-12.

80. Liebowitz MR. Pharmacotherapy of social anxiety disorder. *J Clin Psychiatry*. 1993;54(suppl 12):31-35.

81. Marks IM, Mathews AM. Brief standard self-rating for phobic patients. *Behav Res Ther*. 1979;17:263-267.

82. Mancini C, Van Ameringen M. Paroxetine in social anxiety disorder. *J Clin Psychiatry*. 1996;57:519-522.

83. Stein MB, Liebowitz MR, Lydiard RB, Pitts CD, Bushnell W, Gergee I. Paroxetine treatment of generalized social anxiety disorder: a randomized, double-blind, placebo-controlled study. *JAMA*. 1998;280:708-713.

84. Stein MB, Chartier MJ, Hazen AL. Paroxetine in the treatment of generalized social anxiety disorder: open-label treatment and double-blind, placebo-controlled discontinuation. *J Clin Psychopharmacol*. 1996;16:218-222.

85. Van Ameringen M, Mancini C, Streiner DL. Fluoxetine efficacy in social anxiety disorder. *J Clin Psychiatry*. 1993;54:27-32.

86. Liebowitz MR, Schneier F, Campeas R, et al. Phenelzine vs atenolol in social anxiety disorder: a placebo-controlled comparison. *Arch Gen Psychiatry*. 1992;49:290-300.

87. Davidson JRT, Tupler LA, Potts NLS. Treatment of social anxiety disorder with benzodiazepines. *J Clin Psychiatry*. 1994;55(suppl 6):28-32.

88. Simon GE, VonKorff M, Barlow W. Health care costs of primary care patients with recognized depression. *Arch Gen Psychiatry*. 1995; 52:850-856.

89. Unützer J, Patrick DL, Simon G, et al. Depressive symptoms and the cost of health services in HMO patients aged 65 years and older: a 4-year prospective study. *JAMA*. 1997;277:1618-1623.

90. Depression Guideline Panel. *Depression in Primary Care: Volume 1. Treatment of Major Depression. Clinical Practice Guideline, Number 5.* Rockville, MD: US Department of Health and Human Services, Public Health Service, Agency for Health Care Policy and Research. AHCPR Publication No 93-0551. April 1993.

91. Hirschfeld RMA, Keller MB, Panico S, et al. The National Depressive and Manic-Depressive Association consensus statement on the under-treatment of depression. *JAMA*. 1997;277:333-340.

92. Katon W, Schulberg H. Epidemiology of depression in primary care. *Gen Hosp Psychiatry*. 1992;14:237-247.

93. American Psychiatric Association. Practice guideline for major depressive disorder in adults. *Am J Psychiatry*. 1993;150(April suppl):1-26.

94. Musselman DL, DeBattista C, Nathan KI, Kitts CD, Schatzberg AF, Nemeroff CB. Biology of mood disorders. In: Schatzberg AF, Nemeroff CB, eds. *Textbook of Psychopharmacology*. 2nd ed. Washington, DC: American Psychiatric Press Inc; 1998:549-588.

95. Nemeroff CB. The neurobiology of depression. *Sci Am*. 1998; June: 43-49.

96. DeWester JN. Recognizing and treating the patient with somatic manifestations of depression. *J Fam Pract*. 1996;43(suppl):S3-S15.

97. Gerber PE, Barrett JE, Barrett JA, et al. The relationship of presenting physical complaints to depressive symptoms in primary care patients. *J Gen Intern Med*. 1992;7:170-173.

98. Lyness JM, Noel TK, Cox C, King DA, Conwell Y, Caine ED. Screening for depression in elderly primary care patients: a comparison of the Center for Epidemiologic Studies-Depression Scale and the Geriatric Depression Scale. *Arch Intern Med*. 1997;157:449-454.

99. Mulrow CD, Williams JW Jr, Gerety MB, Ramirez G, Montiel OM, Kerber C. Case-finding instruments for depression in primary care settings. *Ann Intern Med*. 1995;122:913-921.

100. Spitzer RL, Williams JBW, Kroenke K, et al. Utility of a new procedure for diagnosing mental disorders in primary care: the PRIME-MS 1000 study. *JAMA*. 1994;272:1749-1756.

101. Hirschfeld RMA, Russell JM. Assessment and treatment of suicidal patients. *N Engl J Med*. 1997;337:910-915.

102. Evans DA, Staab J, Ward H, et al. Depression in the medically ill: management considerations. *Depression and Anxiety*. 1996/1997;4:199-208.

103. Charney DS, Berman RM, Miller HL. Treatment of depression. In: Schatzberg AF, Nemeroff CB, eds. *Textbook of Psychopharmacology*. 2nd ed. Washington, DC: American Psychiatric Press Inc; 1998:705-731.

104. Depression Guideline Panel. *Depression in Primary Care: Volume 2. Treatment of Major Depression. Clinical Practice Guideline, Number 5.* Rockville, MD: US Department of Health and Human Services, Public Health Service, Agency for Health Care Policy and Research. AHCPR Publication No 93-0551. April 1993.

105. Quitkin FM, McGrath PJ, Stewart JW, et al. Chronologic milestones to guide drug change: when should clinicians switch antidepressants? *Arch Gen Psychiatry*. 1996;53:785-792.

106. Rush AJ. Depression in primary care: detection, diagnosis, and treatment. *Am Fam Physician*. 1993;47:1776-1788.

107. Committee on Adolescent Health Care. ACOG committee opinion. Prevention of adolescent suicide. *Int J Gynaecol Obstet*. 1997;60:83-85.

108. Bostic JQ, Wilens T, Spencer T, Biederman J. Juvenile mood disorders and office pharmacology. *Pediatr Clin North Am*. 1997;44:1487-1503.

109. Kovacs M, Devlin B. Internalizing disorders in childhood. *J Child Psychol Psychiatry*. 1998;39:47-63.

110. Post D, Carr C, Weigand J. Teenagers: mental health and psychological issues. *Prim Care*. 1998;25:181-192.

111. Keller MB, Ryan ND, Birmaher B, et al. Paroxetine and imipramine in the treatment of adolescent depression. Presented at American Psychiatric Association Annual Meeting; May 30-June 4, 1998; Toronto, Ontario, Canada.

112. Reynolds CF III, Zubenko GS, Pollock BG, et al. Depression in late life. *Curr Opin Psychiatry*. 1994;7:18-21.

113. Koenig HG, George LK, Meador KG. Use of antidepressants by nonpsychiatrists in the treatment of medically ill hospitalized depressed elderly patients. *Am J Psychiatry*. 1997;154:1369-1375.

114. Penninx BWJH, Guralnik JM, Ferrucci L, Simonsick EM, Deeg DJH, Wallace RB. Depressive symptoms and physical decline in community-dwelling older persons. *JAMA*. 1998;279:1720-1726.

115. Pitts CD, Morton NH, Goodwin W, Gergel IP. Paroxetine in the treatment of depression in elderly patients (abstract). Presented at American Psychiatric Association Annual Meeting; May 30-June 4, 1998; Toronto, Ontario, Canada.

116. Ferentz KS. Recognizing and treating dysthymia in the primary care patient. In: Ferentz KS, ed. Depression in the primary care patient. Minneapolis, MN: Healthcare Information Programs, McGraw Hill Healthcare Publications Group, 1995; December:13-20 (Postgraduate Medicine Special Report).

117. American Psychiatric Association. Practice guideline for the treatment of patients with bipolar disorder. *Am J Psychiatry.* 1994;151(December suppl):1-36.

118. Gelenberg AJ, Hopkins HS. Report on efficacy of treatments for bipolar disorder. *Psychopharmacol Bull.* 1993;29:447-456.

119. Kahn DA, Carpenter D, Docherty JP, Frances A. Treatment of bipolar disorder. Expert Consensus Guidelines Series. *J Clin Psychiatry.* 1996; 57(suppl 12A):1-88.

120. Dubovsky SL, Buzan RD. Novel alternatives and supplements to lithium and anticonvulsants for bipolar affective disorders. *J Clin Psychiatry.* 1997;58:224-242.

121. Sachs GS. Treatment-resistant bipolar depression. *Psychiatr Clin North Am.* 1996;19:215-236.

122. Schou M. Forty years of lithium treatment. *Arch Gen Psychiatry.* 1997; 54:9-13.

123. Srisurapanont M, Yatham LN, Zis AP. Treatment of acute bipolar depression: a review of the literature. *Can J Psychiatry.* 1995;40:533-544.

124. Kalin NH. Management of the depressive component of bipolar disorder. *Depression and Anxiety.* 1996/1997;4:190-198.

125. Altshuler LL, Post RM, Leverich GS, Mikalauskas K, Rosoff A, Ackerman L. Antidepressant-induced mania and cycle acceleration: a controversy revisited. *Am J Psychiatry.* 1995;152:1130-1138.

126. Wehr TA, Goodwin FK. Can antidepressants cause mania and worsen the course of affective illness? *Am J Psychiatry.* 1987;144:1403-1411.

127. Stoll AL, Mayer PV, Kolbrener M, et al. Antidepressant-associated mania: a controlled comparison with spontaneous mania. *Am J Psychiatry.* 1994;151:1642-1645.

128. Bowden CL. Treatment of bipolar disorder. In: Schatzberg AF, Nemeroff CB, eds. *Textbook of Psychopharmacology.* 2nd ed. Washington, DC: American Psychiatric Press Inc; 1998:733-745.

129. Simon GE, VonKorff M. Prevalence, burden, and treatment of insomnia in primary care. *Am J Psychiatry.* 1997;154:1417-1423.

130. Kupfer DJ, Reynolds CF III. Management of insomnia. *N Engl J Med.* 1997;336:341-346.

131. Farney RJ, Walker JM. Office management of common sleep-wake disorders. *Med Clin North Am.* 1995;79:391-414.

132. Morin CM, Culbert JP, Schwartz SM. Nonpharmacological interventions for insomnia: a meta-analysis of treatment efficacy. *Am J Psychiatry.* 1994;151:1172-1180.

133. Grad RM. Benzodiazepines for insomnia in community-dwelling elderly: a review of benefit and risk. *J Fam Pract.* 1995;41:473-481.

134. Gureje O, Simon GE, Ustun TB, Goldberg DP. Somatization in cross-cultural perspective: a World Health Organization study in primary care. *Am J Psychiatry.* 1997;154:989-995.

135. Kroenke K, Spitzer RL, Williams JBW, et al. Physical symptoms in primary care: predictors of psychiatric disorders and functional impairment. *Arch Fam Med.* 1994;3:774-779.

136. Simon GE, VonKorff M. Somatization and psychiatric disorder in the NIMH Epidemiologic Catchment Area study. *Am J Psychiatry.* 1991;148: 1494-1500.

137. Margo KL, Margo GM. The problem of somatization in family practice. *Am Fam Physician.* 1994;49:1873-1879.

138. Simon GE. Psychiatric disorder and functional somatic symptoms as predictors of health care use. *Psychiatr Med.* 1992;10:49-59.

139. Othmer E, DeSouza C. A screening test for somatization disorder. *Am J Psychiatry.* 1985;142:1146-1149.

140. Smith GR Jr, Rost K, Kashner TM. A trial of the effect of a standardized psychiatric consultation on health outcomes and costs in somatizing patients. *Arch Gen Psychiatry.* 1995;52:238-243.

141. Fleming MF, Barry KL, Manwell LB, Johnson K, London R. Brief physician advice for problem alcohol drinkers: a randomized controlled trial in community-based primary care practices. *JAMA.* 1997;277:1039-1045.

142. Fink A, Hays RD, Moore AA, Beck JC. Alcohol-related problems in older persons: determinants, consequences, and screening. *Arch Intern Med.* 1996;156:1150-1156.

143. Robins LN, Helzer JE, Weissman MM, et al. Lifetime prevalence of specific psychiatric disorders in three sites. *Arch Gen Psychiatry.* 1984;41:949-958.

144. Cornish JW, McNicholas LF, O'Brien CP. Treatment of substance-related disorders. In: Schatzberg AF, Nemeroff CB, eds. *Textbook of Psychopharmacology.* 2nd ed. Washington, DC: American Psychiatric Press Inc; 1998:851-867.

145. Kessler RC, Crum RM, Warner LA, Nelson CB, Schulenber J, Anthony JC. Lifetime co-occurrence of DSM-III-R alcohol abuse and dependence with other psychiatric disorders in the National Comorbidity Survey. *Arch Gen Psychiatry.* 1997;54:313-321.

146. Meyer RE, Berger SP. Biology of psychoactive substance dependence disorders: cocaine, opiates, and ethanol. In: Schatzberg AF, Nemeroff CB, eds. *Textbook of Psychopharmacology.* 2nd ed. Washington, DC: American Psychiatric Press Inc; 1998:649-671.

147. Skinner MH, Thompson DA. Pharmacologic considerations in the treatment of substance abuse. *South Med J.* 1992;85:1207-1219.

148. Ewing JA. Detecting alcoholism: the CAGE questionnaire. *JAMA.* 1984; 252:1905-1907.

149. Selzer ML. The Michigan Alcoholism Screening Test: the quest for a new diagnostic instrument. *Am J Psychiatry.* 1971;127:1653-1658.

150. Isaacson JH, Butler R, Zacharek M, Tzelepis A. Screening with the Alcohol Use Disorders Identification Test (AUDIT) in an inner-city population. *J Gen Intern Med.* 1994;9:550-553.

151. Hoeksema HL, de Bock GH. The value of laboratory tests for the screening and recognition of alcohol abuse in primary care patients. *J Fam Pract.* 1993;37:268-276.

152. Miller NS. Pharmacotherapy in alcoholism. *J Addict Dis.* 1995;12:23-46.

153. Volpicelli JR, Alterman AI, Hayashida M, O'Brien CP. Naltrexone in the treatment of alcohol dependence. *Arch Gen Psychiatry.* 1992;49: 876-880.

154. Tutton CS, Crayton JW. Current pharmacotherapies for cocaine abuse: a review. *J Addict Dis.* 1993;12:109-127.

155. Das G. Cocaine abuse in North America: a milestone in history. *J Clin Pharmacol.* 1993;33:296-310.

156. Kiyatkin EA. Dopamine mechanisms of cocaine addiction. *Int J Neurosci.* 1994;78:75-101.

157. Warner EA. Cocaine abuse. *Ann Intern Med.* 1993;119:226-235.

158. Bartecchi CE, MacKenzie TD, Schrier RW. The human costs of tobacco use (first of two parts). *N Engl J Med.* 1994;330:907-912.

159. Benowitz NL. Cigarette smoking and nicotine addiction. *Med Clin North Am.* 1992;76:415-437.

160. Henningfield JE. Nicotine medications for smoking cessation. *N Engl J Med.* 1995;333:1196-1203.

161. Anonymous. Medical care expenditures attributable to cigarette smoking-United States, 1993. *MMWR Morbid Mortal Wkly Rep.* 1994;43: 469-472.

162. Fiore MC, Bailey WC, Cohen SJ, et al. *Smoking Cessation. Clinical Practice Guideline Number 18.* Rockville, MD: US Department of Health and Human Services, Public Health Service, Agency for Health Care Policy and Research. AHCPR Publication No 96-0692. April 1996.

163. Abramowicz M, ed. Bupropion (Zyban) for smoking cessation. *Med Letter.* 1997;39:77-78.

164. O'Connor PG, Carroll KM, Shi JM, Schottenfeld RS, Kosten TR, Rounsaville BJ. Three methods of opioid detoxification in a primary care setting. *Ann Intern Med.* 1997;127:526-530.

165. Advokat C, Kutlesic V. Pharmacotherapy of the eating disorders: a commentary. *Neurosci Biobehav Rev.* 1995;19:59-66.

166. Shisslak CM, Crago M, Estes LS. The spectrum of eating disturbances. *Int J Eat Disord.* 1995;18:209-219.

167. Casper RC. Biology of eating disorders. In: Schatzberg AF, Nemeroff CB, eds. *Textbook of Psychopharmacology.* 2nd ed. Washington, DC: American Psychiatric Press Inc; 1998:673-689.

168. American Psychiatric Association. Practice guideline for eating disorders. *Am J Psychiatry.* 1993;150:212-228.

169. Brewerton TD. Toward a unified theory of serotonin dysregulation in eating and related disorders. *Psychoneuroendocrinology.* 1995;20: 561-590.

170. Walsh BT, Devlin MJ. The pharmacologic treatment of eating disorders. *Psychiatr Clin North Am.* 1992;15:149-160.

171. Keel PK, Mitchell JE. Outcome in bulimia nervosa. *Am J Psychiatry.* 1997;154:313-321.

172. Walsh BT, Wilson GT, Loeb KL, et al. Medication and psychotherapy in the treatment of bulimia nervosa. *Am J Psychiatry.* 1997;154:523-531.

173. Hughes PL, Wells LA, Cunningham CJ, Ilstrup DM. Treating bulimia with desipramine: a double-blind, placebo-controlled study. *Arch Gen Psychiatry.* 1986;43:182-186.

174. Fluoxetine Bulimia Nervosa Collaborative Study Group. Fluoxetine in the treatment of bulimia nervosa: a multicenter, placebo-controlled, double-blind trial. *Arch Gen Psychiatry.* 1992;49:139-147.

175. Keefover RW. The clinical epidemiology of Alzheimer's disease. *Neurol Clin.* 1996;14:337-351.

176.   Raskind MA. Management of late-life depression and the noncognitive behavioral disturbances of Alzheimer's disease. *Psychiatr Clin North Am.* 1993;16:815-827.

177.   Small GW. Treatment of Alzheimer's disease: current approaches and promising developments. *Am J Med.* 1998;104(suppl 4A):32S-38S.

178.   American Psychiatric Association. Practice guideline for the treatment of patients with Alzheimer's disease and other dementias of late life. *Am J Psychiatry.* 1997;154(May suppl):1-39.

179.   Evans DA, Funkenstein HH, Albert MS, et al. Prevalence of Alzheimer's disease in a community population of older persons: higher than previously reported. *JAMA.* 1989;262:2551-2556.

180.   Cohen GD. Management of Alzheimer's disease. *Adv Intern Med.* 1995;40:31-67.

181.   Salib E, Hillier V. A case-control study of smoking and Alzheimer's disease. *Int J Geriatr Psychiatry.* 1997;12:295-300.

182.   Sandson TA, Sperling RA, Price BH. Alzheimer's disease: an update. *Compr Ther.* 1995;21:480-485.

183.   Small GW. Neuroimaging and genetic assessment for early detection of Alzheimer's disease. *J Clin Psychiatry.* 1996;57(suppl 14):9-13.

184.   Schneider LS, Tariot PN. Emerging drugs for Alzheimer's disease: mechanisms of action and prospects for cognitive-enhancing medications. *Med Clin North Am.* 1994;78:911-934.

185.   Raskind MA, Peskind ER. Treatment of noncognitive symptoms in Alzheimer's disease and other dementias. In: Schatzberg AF, Nemeroff CB, eds. *Textbook of Psychopharmacology.* 2nd ed. Washington, DC: American Psychiatric Press Inc; 1998:791-801.

186.   McKhann G, Drachman D, Folstein M, Katzman R, Price D, Stadlan EM. Clinical diagnosis of Alzheimer's disease: report of the NINCDS-ADRDA Work Group under the auspices of the Department of Health and Human Services Task Force on Alzheimer's disease. *Neurology.* 1984;34:939-944.

187.   de la Monte SM, Ghanbari K, Frey WH, et al. Characterization of the ADFC-NTP cDNA expression in Alzheimer's disease and measurement of a 41-KD protein in cerebrospinal fluid. *J Clin Invest.* 1997;100:3093-3104.

188.   Knopman DS. The initial recognition and diagnosis of dementia. *Am J Med.* 1998;104(suppl 4A):2S-12S.

189.   Folstein M, Folstein S, McHugh PR. Mini-Mental State: a practical method for grading the cognitive state of patients for the clinician. *J Psychiatr Res.* 1975;12:189-198.

190. Blessed G, Tomlinson BE, Roth M. The association between quantitative measures of dementia and of senile change in the cerebral grey matter of elderly subjects. *Br J Psychiatry.* 1968;114:797-811.

191. Pfeiffer E. A short, portable mental status questionnaire for the assessment of organic brain deficit in elderly patients. *J Am Geriatr Soc.* 1975;23:433-441.

192. Peskind ER. Question and answer session. In: Clinical developments in Alzheimer's disease. *J Clin Psychiatry.* 1996;57(suppl 14):39-44.

193. Sky AJ, Grossberg GT. The use of psychotropic medication in the management of problem behaviors in the patient with Alzheimer's disease. *Med Clin North Am.* 1994;78:811-822.

194. Schneider LS. New therapeutic approaches to Alzheimer's disease. *J Clin Psychiatry.* 1996;57(suppl 14):30-36.

195. Schneider LS, Pollock VE, Lyness SA. A meta-analysis of controlled trials of neuroleptic treatment in dementia. *J Am Geriatr Soc.* 1990;38:553-563.

196. Alexopoulos GS. The treatment of depressed demented patients. *J Clin Psychiatry.* 1996;57(suppl 14):14-20.

197. Gleason RP, Schneider LS. Carbamazepine treatment of agitation in Alzheimer's outpatients refractory to neuroleptics. *J Clin Psychiatry.* 1990;51:115-118.

198. Lemke MR. Effect of carbamazepine on agitation in Alzheimer's inpatients refractory to neuroleptics. *J Clin Psychiatry.* 1995;56:354-357.

199. Tariot PN, Erb R, Leibovici A, et al. Carbamazepine treatment of agitation in nursing home patients with dementia: a preliminary study. *J Am Geriatr Soc.* 1994;42:1160-1166.

200. Mellow AM, Solano-Lopez C, Davis S. Sodium valproate in the treatment of behavioral disturbance in dementia. *J Geriatr Psychiatry Neurol.* 1993;6:205-209.

201. Tariot PN. Treatment strategies for agitation and psychosis in dementia. *J Clin Psychiatry.* 1996;57(suppl 14):21-29.

202. Knable MB, Kleinman JE, Weinberger DR. Neurobiology of schizophrenia. In: Schatzberg AF, Nemeroff CB, eds. *Textbook of Psychopharmacology.* 2nd ed. Washington, DC: American Psychiatric Press Inc; 1998:589-607.

203. American Psychiatric Association. Practice guideline for the treatment of patients with schizophrenia. *Am J Psychiatry.* 1997;154(suppl):1-63.

204. Kapur S, Remington G. Serotonin-dopamine interaction and its relevance to schizophrenia. *Am J Psychiatry.* 1996;153:466-476.

205. Keith SJ. Pharmacologic advances in the treatment of schizophrenia (editorial). *N Engl J Med*. 1997;337:851-852.

206. Buckley PF, Meltzer HY. Treatment of schizophrenia. In: Schatzberg AF, Nemeroff CB, eds. *Textbook of Psychopharmacology*. 1st ed. Washington, DC: American Psychiatric Press, Inc; 1995:615-639.

207. Meltzer HY, Fatemi SH. Treatment of schizophrenia. In: Schatzberg AF, Nemeroff CB, eds. *Textbook of Psychopharmacology*. 2nd ed. Washington, DC: American Psychiatric Press Inc; 1998:747-774.

208. Falloon IRH, Boyd JL, McGill CW, et al. Family management in the prevention of morbidity of schizophrenia. *Arch Gen Psychiatry*. 1985;42:887-896.

209. McEvoy JP, Weiden PJ, Smith TE, Carpenter D, Kahn DA, Frances A. Treatment of schizophrenia. Expert Consensus Guidelines Series. *J Clin Psychiatry*. 1996;57(suppl 12B):1-58.

210. Meltzer HY, Lee MA, Ranjan R. Recent advances in the pharmacotherapy of schizophrenia. *Acta Psychiatr Scand*. 1994;90(suppl 384):95-101.

211. Potter WZ, Majni HK, Rudorfer MV. Tricyclics and tetracyclics. In: Schatzberg AF, Nemeroff CB, eds. *Textbook of Psychopharmacology*. 1st ed. Washington, DC: American Psychiatric Press Inc; 1995:141-160.

212. Schatzberg AF, Cole JO, DeBattista D. *Manual of Clinical Psychopharmacology*. 3rd ed. Washington, DC: American Psychiatric Press Inc; 1997.

213. Nemeroff CB, DeVane CL, Pollock BG. Newer antidepressants and the cytochrome P450 system. *Am J Psychiatry*. 1996;153:311-320.

214. de Jonghe F, Swinkels JA. The safety of antidepressants. *Drugs*. 1992;43(suppl 2):40-47.

215. Roose SP, Laghrissi-Thode F, Kennedy JS, et al. Comparison of paroxetine and nortriptyline in depressed patients with ischemic heart disease. *JAMA*. 1998;279:287-291.

216. Cohen LJ. Rational drug use in the treatment of depression. *Pharmacotherapy*. 1997;17:45-61.

217. Kilts CD. Recent pharmacologic advances in antidepressant therapy. *Am J Med*. 1994;97(suppl 6A):3S-12S.

218. DeVane CL. Pharmacokinetics of the newer antidepressants: clinical relevance. *Am J Med*. 1994;97(suppl 6A):13S-23S.

219. Noble S, Benfield P. Citalopram: a review of its pharmacology, clinical efficacy, and tolerability in the treatment of depression. *CNS Drugs*. 1997;5:410-431.

220. Andrews JM, Nemeroff CB. Contemporary management of depression. *Am J Med.* 1994;97(suppl 6A):24S-32S.

221. Gram LF. Fluoxetine. *N Engl J Med.* 1994;331:1354-1361.

222. Holliday SM, Plosker GL. Paroxetine: a review of its pharmacology, therapeutic use in depression, and therapeutic potential in diabetic nephropathy. *Drugs Aging.* 1993;3:278-299.

223. Murdoch D, McTavish D. Sertraline: a review of its pharmacodynamic and pharmacokinetic properties, and therapeutic potential in depression and obsessive-compulsive disorder. *Drugs.* 1992;44:604-624.

224. Ware MR. Fluvoxamine: a review of the controlled trials in depression. *J Clin Psychiatry.* 1997;58(suppl 5):15-23.

225. Wilde MI, Plosker GL, Benfield P. Fluvoxamine: an updated review of its pharmacology and therapeutic use in depressive illness. *Drugs.* 1993;46:895-924.

226. Centorrino F, Baldessarini RJ, Frankenburg FR, Kardo J, Volpicelli SA, Flood JG. Serum levels of clozapine and norclozapine in patients treated with selective serotonin reuptake inhibitors. *Am J Psychiatry.* 1996; 153:820-822.

227. Grundemar L, Wohlfart B, Lagerstedt C, Bengtsson F, Eklundh G. Symptoms and signs of severe citalopram overdose (letter). *Lancet.* 1997;349:1602.

228. Öström M, Eriksson A, Thorson J, Spigset O. Fatal overdose with citalopram. *Lancet.* 1996;348:339-340.

229. Amsterdam JD, Hornig-Rohan M, Maislin G. Efficacy of alprazolam in reducing fluoxetine-induced jitteriness in patients with major depression. *J Clin Psychiatry.* 1994;55:394-400.

230. Modell JG, Katholi CR, Modell JD, DePalma RL. Comparative sexual side effects of bupropion, fluoxetine, paroxetine, and sertraline. *Clin Pharmacol Ther.* 1997;61:476-487.

231. Berk M, Acton M. Citalopram-associated clitoral priapism: a case series. *Int Clin Psychopharmacol.* 1997;12:121-122.

232. Elmore JL, Quattlebaum JT. Female sexual stimulation during antidepressant treatment. *Pharmacotherapy.* 1997;17:612-616.

233. Wisner KL, Perel JM, Findling RL. Antidepressant treatment during breast-feeding. *Am J Psychiatry.* 1996;153:1132-1137.

234. Lejoyeux M, Adès J. Antidepressant discontinuation: a review of the literature. *J Clin Psychiatry.* 1997;58(suppl 7):11-16.

235. Einbinder E. Fluoxetine withdrawal? (letter). *Am J Psychiatry.* 1995; 152:1235.

236. Salzman C. Monoamine oxidase inhibitors and atypical antidepressants. *Clin Geriatr Med.* 1992;8:335-348.

237. Krishnan KRR. Monoamine oxidase inhibitors. In: Schatzberg AF, Nemeroff CB, eds. *Textbook of Psychopharmacology.* 2nd ed. Washington, DC: American Psychiatric Press Inc; 1998:239-249.

238. Quitkin F, Rifkin A, Klein DF. Monoamine oxidase inhibitors: a review of antidepressant effectiveness. *Arch Gen Psychiatry.* 1979;36: 749-760.

239. Gardner DM, Shulman KI, Walker SE, Tailor SAN. The making of a user-friendly MAOI diet. *J Clin Psychiatry.* 1996;57:99-104.

240. Ascher JA, Cole JO, Colin J-N, et al. Bupropion: a review of its mechanism of antidepressant activity. *J Clin Psychiatry.* 1995;56:395-401.

241. Golden RN, Dawkins K, Nicholas L, Bebchuck JM. Trazodone, nefazodone, bupropion, and mirtazapine. In: Schatzberg AF, Nemeroff CB, eds. *Textbook of Psychopharmacology.* 2nd ed. Washington, DC: American Psychiatric Press Inc; 1998:251-269.

242. Roose SP, Dalack GW, Glassman AH, Woodring S, Walsh TB, Giardina EGV. Cardiovascular effects of bupropion in depressed patients with heart disease. *Am J Psychiatry.* 1991;148:512-516.

243. James WA, Lippmann S. Bupropion: overview and prescribing guidelines in depression. *South Med J.* 1991;84:222-224.

244. Stimmel GL, Dopheide JA, Stahl SM. Mirtazapine: an antidepressant with noradrenergic and specific serotonergic effects. *Pharmacotherapy.* 1997;17:10-21.

245. Abramowicz M, ed. Mirtazapine: a new antidepressant. *Med Letter.* 1996;38:113-114.

246. Davis R, Whittington R, Bryson HM. Nefazodone: a review of its pharmacology and clinical efficacy in the management of major depression. *Drugs.* 1997;53:608-636.

247. Feighner JP, Boyer WF. Overview of USA controlled trials of trazodone in clinical depression. *Psychopharmacology.* 1988;95:S50-S53.

248. Haria M, Fitton A, McTavish D. Trazodone: a review of its pharmacology, therapeutic use in depression, and therapeutic potential in other disorders. *Drugs Aging.* 1994;4:331-355.

249. Brogden RN, Heel RC, Speight TM, Avery GS. Trazodone: a review of its pharmacological properties and therapeutic use in depression and anxiety. *Drugs.* 1981;21:401-429.

250. Fabre LF. United States experience and perspectives with trazodone. *Clin Neuropharmacol.* 1989;12(suppl 1):S11-S17.

251. Holliday SM, Benfield P. Venlafaxine: a review of its pharmacology and therapeutic potential in depression. *Drugs.* 1995;49:280-294.

252. Augustin BG, Cold JA, Jann MW. Venlafaxine and nefazodone, two pharmacologically distinct antidepressants. *Pharmacotherapy.* 1997;17: 511-530.

253. Feighner JP. The role of venlafaxine in rational antidepressant therapy. *J Clin Psychiatry.* 1994;55(suppl A):62-68.

254. Thase ME, et al, for the Venlafaxine XR 209 Study Group. Efficacy and tolerability of once-daily venlafaxine extended release (XR) in outpatients with major depression. *J Clin Psychiatry.* 1997;58:393-398.

255. Lenox RH, Manji HK. Lithium. In: Schatzberg AF, Nemeroff CB, eds. *Textbook of Psychopharmacology.* 2nd ed. Washington, DC: American Psychiatric Press Inc; 1998:379-429.

256. Gershon S, Soares JC. Current therapeutic profile of lithium (commentary). *Arch Gen Psychiatry.* 1997;54:16-20.

257. Heit S, Nemeroff CB. Lithium augmentation of antidepressants in treatment-refractory depression. *J Clin Psychiatry.* 1998;59(suppl 6): 28-34.

258. Keck PE Jr, McElroy SL. Antiepileptic drugs. In: Schatzberg AF, Nemeroff CB, eds. *Textbook of Psychopharmacology.* 2nd ed. Washington, DC: American Psychiatric Press Inc; 1998:431-454.

259. Bowden CL, Brugger AM, Swann AC, et al, for the Depakote Mania Study Group. Efficacy of divalproex versus lithium and placebo in the treatment of mania. *JAMA.* 1994;271:918-924.

260. Ballenger JC. Benzodiazepines. In: Schatzberg AF, Nemeroff CB, eds. *Textbook of Psychopharmacology.* 2nd ed. Washington, DC: American Psychiatric Press Inc; 1998:271-286.

261. Shader RI, Greenblatt DJ. Use of benzodiazepines in anxiety disorders. *N Engl J Med.* 1993;328:1398-1405.

262. Lader M. Rebound insomnia and newer hypnotics. *Psychopharmacology.* 1992;108:248-255.

263. Ninan PT, Cole JO, Yonkers KA. Nonbenzodiazepine anxiolytics. In: Schatzberg AF, Nemeroff CB, eds. *Textbook of Psychopharmacology.* 2nd ed. Washington, DC: American Psychiatric Press Inc; 1998:287-300.

264. Rickels K, Amsterdam J, Clary C, et al. Buspirone in depressed outpatients: a controlled study. *Psychopharmacol Bull.* 1990;26:163-167.

265. Kivistö KT, Lamberg TS, Kantola T, Neuvonen PJ. Plasma buspirone concentrations are greatly increased by erythromycin and itraconazole. *Clin Pharmacol Ther.* 1997;62:348-354.

266. Nishino S, Mignot E, Dement WC. Sedative-hypnotics. In: Schatzberg AF, Nemeroff CB, eds. *Textbook of Psychopharmacology*. 1st ed. Washington, DC: American Psychiatric Press Inc; 1995:405-416.

267. Salvà P, Costa J. Clinical pharmacokinetics and pharmacodynamics of zolpidem: therapeutic implications. *Clin Pharmacokinet*. 1995;29: 142-153.

268. Nowell PD, Mazumdar S, Buysse DJ, Dew MA, Reynolds CF III, Kupfer DJ. Benzodiazepines and zolpidem for chronic insomnia: a meta-analysis of treatment efficacy. *JAMA*. 1997;278:2170-2177.

269. Pies RW. Dose-related sensory distortions with zolpidem (letter). *J Clin Psychiatry*. 1995;56:35.

270. Sánchez LGB, Sanchez JM, Moreno JLL. Dependence and tolerance with zolpidem (letter). *Am J Health Syst Pharm*. 1996;53:2638.

271. Marder SR. Antipsychotic medications. In: Schatzberg AF, Nemeroff CB, eds. *Textbook of Psychopharmacology*. 2nd ed. Washington, DC: American Psychiatric Press Inc; 1998:309-321.

272. Janicak PG. The relevance of clinical pharmacokinetics and therapeutic drug monitoring: anticonvulsant mood stabilizers and antipsychotics. *J Clin Psychiatry*. 1993;54(suppl 9):35-41.

273. Owens MJ, Risch SC. Atypical antipsychotics. In: Schatzberg AF, Nemeroff CB, eds. *Textbook of Psychopharmacology*. 2nd ed. Washington, DC: American Psychiatric Press Inc; 1998:323-348.

274. Abramowicz M, ed. Quetiapine for schizophrenia. *Med Letter*. 1997; 39:117-118.

275. Kane JM. Newer antipsychotic drugs: a review of their pharmacology and therapeutic potential. *Drugs*. 1993;46:585-593.

276. Richelson E. Preclinical pharmacology of neuroleptics: focus on new-generation compounds. *J Clin Psychiatry*. 1996;57(suppl 11):4-11.

277. Casey DE. Side-effect profiles of newer antipsychotic agents. *J Clin Psychiatry*. 1996;57(suppl 11):40-45.

278. Byerly MJ, DeVane CL. Pharmacokinetics of clozapine and risperidone: a review of recent literature. *J Clin Psychopharmacol*. 1996;16:177-187.

279. Ereshefsky L. Pharmacokinetics and drug interactions: update for new antipsychotics. *J Clin Psychiatry*. 1996;57(suppl 11):12-25.

280. Baldessarini RJ, Frankenburg FR. Clozapine: a novel antipsychotic agent. *N Engl J Med*. 1991;324:746-754.

281. Kane M, Honigfeld G, Singer J, Meltzer H, and the Clozaril Collaborative Study Group. Clozapine for the treatment-resistant schizophrenic: a double-blind comparison with chlorpromazine. *Arch Gen Psychiatry.* 1988;45:789-796.

282. Calabrese JR, Kimmel SE, Woyshville MJ, et al. Clozapine for treatment-refractory mania. *Am J Psychiatry.* 1996;153:759-764.

283. Dalkilic A, Grosch WN. Neuroleptic malignant syndrome following initiation of clozapine therapy (letter). *Am J Psychiatry.* 1997;154:881-882.

284. Fulton B, Goa KL. Olanzapine: a review of its pharmacological properties and therapeutic efficacy in the management of schizophrenia and related psychoses. *Drugs.* 1997;53:281-298.

285. Abramowicz M, ed. Olanzapine for schizophrenia. *Med Letter.* 1997; 38:5-6.

286. Tollefson GD, Beasley CM Jr, Tran PV, et al. Olanzapine versus haloperidol in the treatment of schizophrenia and schizoaffective and schizophreniform disorders: results of an international collaborative trial. *Am J Psychiatry.* 1997;154:457-465.

287. Tran PV, Dellva MA, Tollefson GD, Beasley CM Jr, Potvin JH, Keisler GM. Extrapyramidal symptoms and tolerability of olanzapine versus haloperidol in the acute treatment of schizophrenia. *J Clin Psychiatry.* 1997;58:205-211.

288. Small JG, Hirsch SR, Arvanitis LA, Miller BG, Link CGG, and the Seroquel Study Group. Quetiapine in patients with schizophrenia: a high- and low-dose, double-blind comparison with placebo. *Arch Gen Psychiatry.* 1997;54:549-557.

289. Grant S, Fitton A. Risperidone: a review of its pharmacology and therapeutic potential in the treatment of schizophrenia. *Drugs.* 1994;48: 253-273.

290. Stanilla JK, Simpson GM. Treatment of extrapyramidal side effects. In: Schatzberg AF, Nemeroff CB, eds. *Textbook of Psychopharmacology.* 2nd ed. Washington, DC: American Psychiatric Press Inc; 1998:349-375.

291. Klett CJ, Caffey E Jr. Evaluating the long-term need for antiparkinson drugs by chronic schizophrenics. *Arch Gen Psychiatry.* 1972;26: 374-379.

292. Blaisdell GD. Akathisia: a comprehensive review and treatment summary. *Psychopharmacol Bull.* 1994;27:139-146.

293. Rosen WG, Mohs RC, Davis KL. A new rating scale for Alzheimer's disease. *Am J Psychiatry.* 1984;141:1356-1364.

294. Davis KL, Thal LJ, Gamzu ER, et al, for the Tacrine Collaborative Study Group. A double-blind, placebo-controlled multicenter study of tacrine for Alzheimer's disease. *N Engl J Med.* 1992;327:1253-1259.

295. Farlow M, Gracon SI, Hershey LA, Lewis KW, Sadowsky CH, Dolan-Ureno J, for the Tacrine Study Group. A controlled trial of tacrine in Alzheimer's disease. *JAMA.* 1992;268:2523-2529.

296. Knapp MJ, Knopman DS, Solomon PR, Pendlebury WW, Davis CS, Gracon SI, for the Tacrine Study Group. A 30-week, randomized controlled trial of high-dose tacrine in patients with Alzheimer's disease. *JAMA.* 1994;271:985-991.

297. Ohnishi A, Mihara M, Kamakura H, et al. Comparison of the pharmacokinetics of E2020, a new compound for Alzheimer's disease, in healthy young and elderly subjects. *J Clin Pharmacol.* 1993;33:1086-1091.

298. Rogers SL, Friedhoff LT. The efficacy and safety of donepezil in patients with Alzheimer's disease: results of a US multicenter, randomized, double-blind, placebo-controlled trial. The Donepezil Study Group. *Dementia.* 1996;7:293-303.

299. Rogers SL, Doody RS, Mohs RC, Friedhoff LT, and the Donepezil Study Group. Donepezil improves cognition and global function in Alzheimer disease: a 15-week, double-blind, placebo-controlled study. *Arch Intern Med.* 1998;158:1021-1031.

300. Rogers SL, Doody R, Mohs R, Freidhoff LT. E2020 produces both clinical global and cognitive test improvement in patients with mild to moderately severe Alzheimer's disease: results of a 30-week phase III trial (abstract S14.001). *Neurology.* 1996;46:A217.

301. Sano M, Ernseto C, Thomas RG, et al, for the Alzheimer's Disease Cooperative Study. A controlled trial of selegiline, alpha-tocopherol, or both as treatment for Alzheimer's disease. *N Engl J Med.* 1997;336:1216-1222.

302. Schneider LS, Tariot PN, Goldstein B. Therapy with *l*-deprenyl (selegiline) and relation to abuse liability. *Clin Pharmacol Ther.* 1994;56:750-756.

303. Tariot PN, Sunderland T, Weingartner H, et al. Cognitive effects of L-deprenyl in Alzheimer's disease. *Psychopharmacology.* 1987;91:489-495.

304. Fawcett J, Busch KA. Stimulants in psychiatry. In: Schatzberg AF, Nemeroff CB, eds. *Textbook of Psychopharmacology.* 2nd ed. Washington, DC: American Psychiatric Press Inc; 1998:503-522.

305. Altshuler LL, Cohen L, Szuba MP, Burt VK, Gitlin M, Mintz J. Pharmacologic management of psychiatric illness during pregnancy: dilemmas and guidelines. *Am J Psychiatry*. 1996;153:592-606.

306. Kulin NA, Pastuszak A, Sage S, et al. Pregnancy outcome following maternal use of the new selective serotonin reuptake inhibitors: a prospective, controlled, multicenter study. *JAMA*. 1998;279:609-610.

307. Platt JE, Freidhoff AJ, Broman SH, Bond RN, Laska E, Lin SP. Effects of prenatal exposure to neuroleptic drugs on children's growth. *Neuropsychopharmacology*. 1988;1:205-212.

308. Stowe ZN, Strader JR Jr, Nemeroff CB. Psychopharmacology during pregnancy and lactation. In: Schatzberg AF, Nemeroff CB, eds. *Textbook of Psychopharmacology*. 2nd ed. Washington, DC: American Psychiatric Press Inc; 1998:979-996.

309. Jensen PN, Olesen OV, Bertelsen A, Linnet K. Citalopram and desmethylcitalopram concentrations in breast milk and in serum of mother and infant. *Ther Drug Monit*. 1997;19:236-239.

310. Suri RA, Altschuler LL, Burt VK, Hendrick VC. Managing psychiatric medications in the breast-feeding woman. *Medscape Women's Health*. 1998;3:1-14. Available at: http://www.medscape.com/Medscape/womens.health/1998/v03.n01/wh3062.suri/wh3062.suri.html. Accessed April 27, 1998.

311. American Academy of Pediatrics Committee on Drugs. The transfer of drugs and other chemicals into human milk. *Pediatrics*. 1994;93:137-150.

312. Cadieux RJ. Geriatric psychopharmacology: a primary care challenge. *Postgrad Med*. 1993;93:281-301.

313. Salzman C, Satlin A, Burrows AB. Geriatric psychopharmacology. In: Schatzberg AF, Nemeroff CB, eds. *Textbook of Psychopharmacology*. 2nd ed. Washington, DC: American Psychiatric Press Inc; 1998:961-977.

Appendices

TABLE OF DRUGS USED IN PSYCHIATRY

Generic Name	Trade Names (Examples)
ACETYLCHOLINESTERASE INHIBITORS (Dementia Cognitive Enhancers)	
donepezil	Aricept
tacrine HCl	Cognex
ANTIANXIETY DRUGS	
Antihistamines	
diphenhydramine	Benadryl
hydroxyzine	Atarax, Vistaril
Benzodiazepines	
alprazolam	Xanax
chlordiazepoxide	Librium (and others)
clonazepam	Klonopin
clorazepate	Tranxene
diazepam	Valium
halazepam	Paxipam
lorazepam	Ativan
oxazepam	Serax
prazepam	Centrax
Azaspirodione	
buspirone hydrochloride	BuSpar
ANTIDEPRESSANT DRUGS	
Monoamine oxidase inhibitors	
isocarboxazid	Marplan
phenelzine	Nardil
selegiline, L-deprenyl	Eldepryl
tranylcypromine sulfate	Parnate
Tricyclics and similar compounds	
amitriptyline	Amitril, Elavil, Endep
amoxapine	Asendin
clomipramine	Anafranil
desipramine	Norpramin, Pertofrane
doxepin	Adapin, Sinequan

TABLE OF DRUGS USED IN PSYCHIATRY (continued)

Generic Name	Trade Names (Examples)
Tricyclics and similar compounds (continued)	
imipramine	Tofranil (and others)
maprotiline	Ludiomil
nortriptyline	Aventyl, Pamelor
protriptyline	Vivactil
trimipramine	Surmontil
Selective norepinephrine reuptake inhibitor	
reboxetine	Edronax (FDA approval pending 1999)
Selective serotonin reuptake inhibitors	
citalopram	Celexa
fluoxetine	Prozac
fluvoxamine	Luvox
paroxetine	Paxil
sertraline	Zoloft
5-HT$_2$ antagonists	
nefazodone	Serzone
trazodone	Desyrel
Selective serotonin-norepinephrine reuptake inhibitor	
venlafaxine	Effexor (XR)
Atypical antidepressants	
bupropion	Wellbutrin (SR)
mirtazapine	Remeron
HYPNOTICS	
Nonbenzodiazepine hypnotics	
chloral hydrate	Noctec
diphenhydramine	Benadryl
ethchlorvynol	Placidyl
ethinamate	Valmid
glutethimide	Doriden
methyprylon	Noludar
zolpidem	Ambien

TABLE OF DRUGS USED IN PSYCHIATRY (continued)

Generic Name	Trade Names (Examples)
Sedative-hypnotic benzodiazepines	
estazolam	ProSom
flurazepam	Dalmane
quazepam	Doral
temazepam	Restoril
triazolam	Halcion
ANTIMANIC DRUGS	
Lithium salts	
lithium carbonate	Eskalith, Lithane, Lithobid, Lithonate, Lithotabs
lithium citrate	Cibalith-S
ANTICONVULSANT DRUGS	
carbamazepine	Tegretol
gabapentin	Neurontin
lamotrigine	Lamictal
valproic acid	Depakene, Depakote
ANTIPSYCHOTIC DRUGS	
ziprasidone	Zeldax (FDA approval pending 1999)
Benzisoxazole	
risperidone	Risperdal
Butyrophenones	
droperidol	Inapsine
haloperidol	Haldol
Dibenzazepines	
clozapine	Clozaril
loxapine	Daxolin, Loxitane
Dibenzothiazepine	
quetiapine	Seroquel
Dihydroindolone	
molindone	Lidone, Moban

Generic Name	Trade Names (Examples)
Diphenylbutylpiperidine	
pimozide	Orap
Phenothiazines	
Aliphatic	
chlorpromazine	Thorazine
triflupromazine	Vesprin
Piperazine	
acetophenazine	Tindal
fluphenazine	Prolixin, Permitil
perphenazine	Trilafon
trifluoperazine	Stelazine
Piperidine	
mesoridazine	Serentil
piperacetazine	Quide
thioridazine	Mellaril
Thioxanthenes	
chlorprothixene	Taractan
thiothixene	Navane
Thienbenzodiazepine	
olanzapine	Zyprexa

LIEBOWITZ SOCIAL ANXIETY SCALE

(reproduced from reference 80, with permission). © Copyright 1993, Physicians Postgraduate Press.

		Fear	Avoidance
1.	Telephoning in public (P)	_____	_____
2.	Participating in small groups (P)	_____	_____
3.	Eating in public places (P)	_____	_____
4.	Drinking with others in public places (P)	_____	_____
5.	Talking to people in authority (S)	_____	_____
6.	Acting, performing or giving a talk in front of an audience (P)	_____	_____
7.	Going to a party (S)	_____	_____
8.	Working while being observed (P)	_____	_____
9.	Writing while being observed (P)	_____	_____
10.	Calling someone you don't know very well (S)	_____	_____
11.	Talking with people you don't know very well (S)	_____	_____
12.	Meeting strangers (S)	_____	_____
13.	Urinating in a public bathroom (P)	_____	_____
14.	Entering a room when others are already seated (P)	_____	_____
15.	Being the center of attention (S)	_____	_____
16.	Speaking up at a meeting (P)	_____	_____
17.	Taking a test (P)	_____	_____
18.	Expressing a disagreement or disapproval to people you don't know very well (S)	_____	_____
19.	Looking at people you don't know very well in the eyes (S)	_____	_____
20.	Giving a report to a group (P)	_____	_____
21.	Trying to pick up someon (P)	_____	_____
22.	Returning goods to a store (S)	_____	_____
23.	Giving a party (S)	_____	_____
24.	Resisting a high pressure salesperson (S)	_____	_____

	Fear	Avoidance
Total Score	_____	_____
Performance (P) subscores	_____	_____
Social (S) subscores	_____	_____

Fear or anxiety: 0 = none,   1 = mild,   2 = moderate,   3 = severe.

Avoidance: 0 = never (0%),   1 = occasionally (1% to 33%),   2 = often (33% to 67%),   3 = usually (67% to 100%).

P = performance situation;   S = social situation.

M.I.N.I.

MINI INTERNATIONAL NEUROPSYCHIATRIC INTERVIEW

English Version 5.0.0

DSM-IV

USA: **D. Sheehan, J. Janavs, R. Baker, K. Harnett-Sheehan, E. Knapp, M. Sheehan**
University of South Florida - Tampa

FRANCE: **Y. Lecrubier, E. Weiller, T. Hergueta, P. Amorim, L. I. Bonora, J. P. Lépine**
Hôpital de la Salpétrière - Paris

M.I.N.I. 5.0.0 (July 1, 1999)

MINI STRUCTURED INTERVIEW (continued)

	MODULES	TIME FRAME	MEETS CRITERIA	DSM-IV	ICD-10
A	MAJOR DEPRESSIVE EPISODE	Current (2 weeks) ☐ / Past ☐		296.20-296.26 Single / 296.30-296.36 Recurrent	F32.x / F33.x
	MDE WITH MELANCHOLIC FEATURES Optional	Current (2 weeks) ☐		296.20-296.26 Single / 296.30-296.36 Recurrent	F32.x / F33.x
B	DYSTHYMIA	Current (Past 2 years) ☐		300.4	F34.1
C	SUICIDALITY	Current (Past Month) ☐ / Risk: ☐ Low ☐ Medium ☐ High			
D	MANIC EPISODE	Current ☐ / Past ☐		296.00-296.06	F30.x-F31.9
	HYPOMANIC EPISODE	Current ☐ / Past ☐		296.80-296.89	F31.8-F31.9/F34.0
E	PANIC DISORDER	Current (Past Month) ☐ / Lifetime ☐		300.01/300.21	F40.01-F41.0
F	AGORAPHOBIA	Current ☐		300.22	F40.00
G	SOCIAL PHOBIA (Social Anxiety Disorder)	Current (Past Month) ☐		300.23	F40.1
H	OBSESSIVE-COMPULSIVE DISORDER	Current (Past Month) ☐		300.3	F42.8
I	POSTTRAUMATIC STRESS DISORDER Optional	Current (Past Month) ☐		309.81	F43.1
J	ALCOHOL DEPENDENCE / ALCOHOL ABUSE	Past 12 Months ☐ / Past 12 Months ☐		303.9 / 305.00	F10.2x / F10.1
K	DRUG DEPENDENCE (Non-alcohol) / DRUG ABUSE (Non-alcohol)	Past 12 Months ☐ / Past 12 Months ☐		304.00-.90/305.20-.90 / 304.00-.90/305.20-.90	F11.1-F19.1 / F11.1-F19.1
L	PSYCHOTIC DISORDERS	Lifetime ☐ / Current ☐		295.10-295.90/297.1/ 297.3/293.81/293.82/ 293.89/298.8/298.9	F20.xx-F29
	MOOD DISORDER WITH PSYCHOTIC FEATURES	Current ☐		296.24	F32.3/F33.3
M	ANOREXIA NERVOSA	Current (Past 3 Months) ☐		307.1	F50.0
N	BULIMIA NERVOSA	Current (Past 3 Months) ☐		307.51	F50.2
	ANOREXIA NERVOSA, BINGE EATING/PURGING TYPE	Current ☐		307.1	F50.0
O	GENERALIZED ANXIETY DISORDER	Current (Past 6 Months) ☐		300.02	F41.1
P	ANTISOCIAL PERSONALITY DISORDER Optional	Lifetime ☐		301.7	F60.2

MINI STRUCTURED INTERVIEW (continued)

GENERAL INSTRUCTIONS

The M.I.N.I. was designed as a brief structured interview for the major Axis I psychiatric disorders in DSM-IV and ICD-10. Validation and reliability studies have been done comparing the M.I.N.I. to the SCID-P for DSM-III-R and the CIDI (a structured interview developed by the World Health Organization for lay interviewers for ICD-10). The results of these studies show that the M.I.N.I. has acceptably high validation and reliability scores, but can be administered in a much shorter period of time (mean 18.7 ± 11.6 minutes, median 15 minutes) than the above referenced instruments. It can be used by clinicians, after a brief training session. Lay interviewers require more extensive training.

INTERVIEW:

In order to keep the interview as brief as possible, inform the patient that you will conduct a clinical interview that is more structured than usual, with very precise questions about psychological problems which require a yes or no answer.

GENERAL FORMAT:

The M.I.N.I. is divided into **modules** identified by letters, each corresponding to a diagnostic category.
• At the beginning of each diagnostic module (except for psychotic disorders module), screening question(s) corresponding to the main criteria of the disorder are presented in a gray box.
• At the end of each module, diagnostic box(es) permit the clinician to indicate whether diagnostic criteria are met.

CONVENTIONS:

Sentences written in « normal font » should be read exactly as written to the patient in order to standardize the assessment of diagnostic criteria.

Sentences written in « CAPITALS » should not be read to the patient. They are instructions for the interviewer to assist in the scoring of the diagnostic algorithms.

Sentences written in « bold » indicate the time frame being investigated. The interviewer should read them as often as necessary. Only symptoms occurring during the time frame indicated should be considered in scoring the responses.

Answers with an arrow above them (➡) indicate that one of the criteria necessary for the diagnosis(es) is not met. In this case, the interviewer should go to the end of the module, circle « NO » in all the diagnostic boxes and move to the next module.

When terms are separated by a *slash (/)* the interviewer should read only those symptoms known to be present in the patient (for example, question A4b).

Phrases in (parentheses) are clinical examples of the symptom. These may be read to the patient to clarify the question.

RATING INSTRUCTIONS:

All questions must be rated. The rating is done at the right of each question by circling either Yes or No.

The clinician should be sure that each dimension of the question is taken into account by the patient (for example, time frame, frequency, severity, and/or alternatives).

Symptoms better accounted for by an organic cause or by the use of alcohol or drugs should not be coded positive in the M.I.N.I. The M.I.N.I. Plus has questions that investigate these issues.

For any questions, suggestions, need for a training session, or information about updates of the M.I.N.I., please contact :

David V Sheehan, M.D., M.B.A.
University of South Florida
Institute for Research in Psychiatry
3515 East Fletcher Avenue
Tampa, FL USA 33613-4788
tel : +1 813 974 4544: fax : +1 813 974 4575
e-mail : dsheehan@com1.med.usf.edu

Yves Lecrubier, M.D. / Thierry Hergueta, M.S.
INSERM U302
Hôpital de la Salpétrière
47, boulevard de l'Hôpital
F. 75651 PARIS, FRANCE
tel : +33 (0) 1 42 16 16 59   : fax : +33 (0) 1 45 85 28 00
e-mail : hergueta@ext.jussieu.fr

M.I.N.I. 5.0.0 (July 1, 1999)

3

A. MAJOR DEPRESSIVE EPISODE

(➡ MEANS : GO TO THE DIAGNOSTIC BOXES, CIRCLE NO IN ALL DIAGNOSTIC BOXES, AND MOVE TO THE NEXT MODULE)

A1	Have you been consistently depressed or down, most of the day, nearly every day, for the past two weeks?	NO	YES	1
A2	In the past two weeks, have you been less interested in most things or less able to enjoy the things you used to enjoy most of the time?	NO	YES	2
	IS A1 OR A2 CODED YES?	➡ NO	YES	

A3   Over the past two weeks, when you felt depressed or uninterested:

a	Was your appetite decreased or increased nearly every day? Did your weight decrease or increase without trying intentionally (i.e., by ±5% of body weight or ±8 lbs. or ±3.5 kgs., for a 160 lb./70 kg. person in a month)? IF YES TO EITHER, CODE YES.	NO	YES	3
b	Did you have trouble sleeping nearly every night (difficulty falling asleep, waking up in the middle of the night, early morning wakening or sleeping excessively)?	NO	YES	4
c	Did you talk or move more slowly than normal or were you fidgety, restless or having trouble sitting still almost every day?	NO	YES	5
d	Did you feel tired or without energy almost every day?	NO	YES	6
e	Did you feel worthless or guilty almost every day?	NO	YES	7
f	Did you have difficulty concentrating or making decisions almost every day?	NO	YES	8
g	Did you repeatedly consider hurting yourself, feel suicidal, or wish that you were dead?	NO	YES	9

ARE 3 OR MORE A3 ANSWERS CODED YES? (OR 4 A3
ANSWERS IF A1 OR A2 ARE CODED NO)?

NO	YES
MAJOR DEPRESSIVE *EPISODE CURRENT*	

IF PATIENT HAS CURRENT MAJOR DEPRESSIVE EPISODE CONTINUE TO A4,
OTHERWISE MOVE TO MODULE B :

A4 a   During your lifetime, did you have other periods of two weeks or more when you felt   ➡ NO   YES   10
       depressed or uninterested in most things, and had most of the problems we just talked about?

NO	YES	11
MAJOR DEPRESSIVE *EPISODE PAST*		

   b   Did you ever have an interval of at least 2 months without any depression
       and any loss of interest between 2 episodes of depression?

M.I.N.I. 5.0.0 (July 1, 1999)   4

MINI STRUCTURED INTERVIEW (continued)

MAJOR DEPRESSIVE EPISODE WITH MELANCHOLIC FEATURES (optional)

(➡ MEANS : GO TO THE DIAGNOSTIC BOX, CIRCLE NO, AND MOVE TO THE NEXT MODULE)

IF THE PATIENT CODES POSITIVE FOR A CURRENT MAJOR DEPRESSIVE EPISODE (A4 = YES), EXPLORE THE FOLLOWING:

A6	a	IS A2 CODED YES ?	NO	YES	
	b	During the most severe period of the current depressive episode, did you lose your ability to respond to things that previously gave you pleasure, or cheered you up?	NO	YES	12
		IF NO: When something good happens does it fail to make you feel better, even temporarily?			
		IS EITHER A6a OR A6b CODED YES?	➡ NO	YES	
A7		**Over the past two week period, when you felt depressed and uninterested:**			
	a	Did you feel depressed in a way that is different from the kind of feeling you experience when someone close to you dies?	NO	YES	13
	b	Did you feel regularly worse in the morning, almost every day?	NO	YES	14
	c	Did you wake up at least 2 hours before the usual time of awakening and have difficulty getting back to sleep, almost every day?	NO	YES	15
	d	IS A3c CODED YES (PSYCHOMOTOR RETARDATION OR AGITATION)?	NO	YES	
	e	IS A3a CODED YES (ANOREXIA OR WEIGHT LOSS)?	NO	YES	
	f	Did you feel excessive guilt or guilt out of proportion to the reality of the situation?	NO	YES	16

ARE 3 OR MORE A7 ANSWERS CODED YES?

```
NO        YES

Major Depressive Episode
        with
Melancholic Features
      Current
```

M.I.N.I. 5.0.0 (July 1, 1999)   5

B. DYSTHYMIA

(➡ MEANS : GO TO THE DIAGNOSTIC BOX, CIRCLE NO, AND MOVE TO THE NEXT MODULE)

IF PATIENT'S SYMPTOMS CURRENTLY MEET CRITERIA FOR MAJOR DEPRESSIVE EPISODE, DO NOT EXPLORE THIS MODULE.

B1	Have you felt sad, low or depressed most of the time for the last two years?	➡ NO	YES	17
B2	Was this period interrupted by your feeling OK for two months or more?	NO	➡ YES	18
B3	**During this period of feeling depressed most of the time:**			
a	Did your appetite change significantly?	NO	YES	19
b	Did you have trouble sleeping or sleep excessively?	NO	YES	20
c	Did you feel tired or without energy?	NO	YES	21
d	Did you lose your self-confidence?	NO	YES	22
e	Did you have trouble concentrating or making decisions?	NO	YES	23
f	Did you feel hopeless?	NO	YES	24
	ARE 2 OR MORE B3 ANSWERS CODED YES?	➡ NO	YES	
B4	Did the symptoms of depression cause you significant distress or impair your ability to function at work, socially, or in some other important way?	➡ NO	YES	25

NO	YES
	DYSTHYMIA **CURRENT**

IS B4 CODED YES?

C. SUICIDALITY

In the past month did you:

				Points
C1	Think that you would be better off dead or wish you were dead?	NO	YES	1
C2	Want to harm yourself?	NO	YES	2
C3	Think about suicide?	NO	YES	6
C4	Have a suicide plan?	NO	YES	10
C5	Attempt suicide?	NO	YES	10

In your lifetime:

C6	Did you ever make a suicide attempt?	NO	YES	4

IS AT LEAST 1 OF THE ABOVE CODED YES?

IF YES ADD THE TOTAL NUMBER OF POINTS FOR THE ANSWERS (C1-C6) CHECKED 'YES' AND SPECIFY THE LEVEL OF SUICIDE RISK AS FOLLOWS:

NO		YES
SUICIDE RISK		
CURRENT		
1-5 points	Low	☐
6-8 points	Moderate	☐
≥ 10 points	High	☐

D. (HYPO) MANIC EPISODE

(➡ MEANS : GO TO THE DIAGNOSTIC BOXES, CIRCLE NO IN ALL DIAGNOSTIC BOXES, AND MOVE TO THE NEXT MODULE)

D1 a	Have you ever had a period of time when you were feeling 'up' or 'high' or so full of energy or full of yourself that you got into trouble, or that other people thought you were not your usual self? (Do not consider times when you were intoxicated on drugs or alcohol.) IF PATIENT IS PUZZLED OR UNCLEAR ABOUT WHAT YOU MEAN BY 'UP' OR 'HIGH', CLARIFY AS FOLLOWS: By 'up' or 'high' I mean: having elated mood; increased energy; needing less sleep; having rapid thoughts; being full of ideas; having an increase in productivity, motivation, creativity, or impulsive behavior. IF YES:	NO YES	1
b	Are you currently feeling 'up' or 'high' or full of energy?	NO YES	2
D2 a	Have you ever been persistently irritable, for several days, so that you had arguments or verbal or physical fights, or shouted at people outside your family? Have you or others noticed that you have been more irritable or over reacted, compared to other people, even in situations that you felt were justified? IF YES:	NO YES	3
b	Are you currently feeling persistently irritable?	NO YES	4
	IS D1a OR D2a CODED YES?	➡ NO YES	

D3 IF D1b OR D2b = YES: EXPLORE ONLY CURRENT EPISODE
IF D1b AND D2b = NO: EXPLORE THE MOST SYMPTOMATIC PAST EPISODE

During the times when you felt high, full of energy, or irritable did you:

a	Feel that you could do things others couldn't do, or that you were an especially important person?	NO YES	5
b	Need less sleep (for example, feel rested after only a few hours sleep)?	NO YES	6
c	Talk too much without stopping, or so fast that people had difficulty understanding?	NO YES	7
d	Have racing thoughts?	NO YES	8
e	Become easily distracted so that any little interruption could distract you?	NO YES	9
f	Become so active or physically restless that others were worried about you?	NO YES	10
g	Want so much to engage in pleasurable activities that you ignored the risks or consequences (for example, spending sprees, reckless driving, or sexual indiscretions)?	NO YES	11
	ARE 3 OR MORE D3 ANSWERS CODED YES (OR 4 IF D1a IS NO [PAST EPISODE] OR D1b IS NO [CURRENT EPISODE])?	➡ NO YES	

M.I.N.I. 5.0.0 (July 1, 1999)   8

D4   Did these symptoms last at least a week **and** cause significant problems at home,   NO   YES   12
at work, socially, or at school, **or** were you hospitalized for these problems?

                                      ↓   ↓

                  THE EPISODE EXPLORED WAS A: ☐   ☐
                                                  HYPOMANIC   *MANIC*
                                                  EPISODE   *EPISODE*

IS **D4** CODED NO?

	NO	YES
		(HYPO)MANIC EPISODE

SPECIFY IF THE EPISODE IS CURRENT OR PAST.

CURRENT   ☐
PAST   ☐

IS **D4** CODED YES?

	NO	YES
		MANIC EPISODE

SPECIFY IF THE EPISODE IS CURRENT OR PAST.

CURRENT   ☐
PAST   ☐

M.I.N.I. 5.0.0 (July 1, 1999)

                                          9

E. PANIC DISORDER

(➡ MEANS : CIRCLE NO IN E5 AND SKIP TO F1)

E1	a	Have you, on more than one occasion, had spells or attacks when you **suddenly** felt anxious, frightened, uncomfortable or uneasy, even in situations where most people would not feel that way?	➡ NO	YES	1
	b	Did the spells peak within 10 minutes?	➡ NO	YES	2
E2		At any time in the past, did any of those spells or attacks come on unexpectedly or occur in an unpredictable or unprovoked manner?	➡ NO	YES	3
E3		Have you ever had one such attack followed by a month or more of persistent fear of having another attack, or worries about the consequences of the attack?	NO	YES	4
E4		**During the worst spell that you can remember:**			
	a	Did you have skipping, racing or pounding of your heart?	NO	YES	5
	b	Did you have sweating or clammy hands?	NO	YES	6
	c	Were you trembling or shaking?	NO	YES	7
	d	Did you have shortness of breath or difficulty breathing?	NO	YES	8
	e	Did you have a choking sensation or a lump in your throat?	NO	YES	9
	f	Did you have chest pain, pressure or discomfort?	NO	YES	10
	g	Did you have nausea, stomach problems or sudden diarrhea?	NO	YES	11
	h	Did you feel dizzy, unsteady, lightheaded or faint?	NO	YES	12
	i	Did things around you feel strange, unreal, detached or unfamiliar, or did you feel outside of or detached from part or all of your body?	NO	YES	13
	j	Did you fear that you were losing control or going crazy?	NO	YES	14
	k	Did you fear that you were dying?	NO	YES	15
	l	Did you have tingling or numbness in parts of your body?	NO	YES	16
	m	Did you have hot flushes or chills?	NO	YES	17
E5		ARE BOTH E3 AND 4 OR MORE E4 ANSWERS CODED YES?	NO	YES *PANIC DISORDER LIFETIME*	
E6		IF E5 = NO, ARE 1, 2 OR 3 SYMPTOMS IN E4a-m CODED YES?	NO	YES *LIMITED SYMPTOM ATTACKS CURRENT*	
		IF YES TO E6, SKIP TO **F1**.			
E7		In the past month, did you have such attacks repeatedly (2 or more) followed by persistent fear of having another attack?	NO	YES *PANIC DISORDER CURRENT*	18

M.I.N.I. 5.0.0 (July 1, 1999)   10

F. AGORAPHOBIA

F1	Do you feel anxious or uneasy in places or situations where you might have a panic attack or the panic-like symptoms we just spoke about, or where help might not be available or escape might be difficult: like being in a crowd, standing in a line (queue), when you are alone away from home or alone at home, or when crossing a bridge, traveling in a bus, train or car?	NO YES 19

IF **F1** = NO, CIRCLE NO IN **F2**.

F2	Do you fear these situations so much that you avoid them, or suffer through them, or need a companion to face them?	NO YES 20 *AGORAPHOBIA CURRENT*

IS **F2** (CURRENT AGORAPHOBIA) CODED **NO**

and

IS **E7** (CURRENT PANIC DISORDER) CODED **YES**?

> **NO   YES**
>
> ***PANIC DISORDER***
> ***without Agoraphobia***
> ***CURRENT***

IS **F2** (CURRENT AGORAPHOBIA) CODED **YES**

and

IS **E7** (CURRENT PANIC DISORDER) CODED **YES**?

> **NO   YES**
>
> ***PANIC DISORDER***
> ***with Agoraphobia***
> ***CURRENT***

IS **F2** (CURRENT AGORAPHOBIA) CODED **YES**

and

IS **E5** (PANIC DISORDER LIFETIME) CODED **NO**?

> **NO   YES**
>
> ***AGORAPHOBIA, CURRENT***
> ***without history of***
> ***Panic Disorder***

G. SOCIAL PHOBIA (Social Anxiety Disorder)

(➡ MEANS : GO TO THE DIAGNOSTIC BOX, CIRCLE NO AND MOVE TO THE NEXT MODULE)

G1	In the past month, were you fearful or embarrassed being watched, being the focus of attention, or fearful of being humiliated? This includes things like speaking in public, eating in public or with others, writing while someone watches, or being in social situations.	➡ NO	YES	1
G2	Is this fear excessive or unreasonable?	➡ NO	YES	2
G3	Do you fear these situations so much that you avoid them or suffer through them?	➡ NO	YES	3
G4	Does this fear disrupt your normal work or social functioning or cause you significant distress?	NO	YES	4

SOCIAL PHOBIA
(Social Anxiety Disorder)
CURRENT

H. OBSESSIVE-COMPULSIVE DISORDER

(➡ MEANS : GO TO THE DIAGNOSTIC BOX, CIRCLE NO AND MOVE TO THE NEXT MODULE)

H1	In the past month, have you been bothered by recurrent thoughts, impulses, or images that were unwanted, distasteful, inappropriate, intrusive, or distressing? (For example, the idea that you were dirty, contaminated or had germs, or fear of contaminating others, or fear of harming someone even though you didn't want to, or fearing you would act on some impulse, or fear or superstitions that you would be responsible for things going wrong, or obsessions with sexual thoughts, images or impulses, or hoarding, collecting, or religious obsessions.) (DO NOT INCLUDE SIMPLY EXCESSIVE WORRIES ABOUT REAL LIFE PROBLEMS. DO NOT INCLUDE OBSESSIONS DIRECTLY RELATED TO EATING DISORDERS, SEXUAL DEVIATIONS, PATHOLOGICAL GAMBLING, OR ALCOHOL OR DRUG ABUSE BECAUSE THE PATIENT MAY DERIVE PLEASURE FROM THE ACTIVITY AND MAY WANT TO RESIST IT ONLY BECAUSE OF ITS NEGATIVE CONSEQUENCES.)	NO ➡to H4	YES	1
H2	Did they keep coming back into your mind even when you tried to ignore or get rid of them?	NO ➡to H4	YES	2
H3	Do you think that these obsessions are the product of your own mind and that they are not imposed from the outside?	NO	YES [obsessions]	3
H4	In the past month, did you do something repeatedly without being able to resist doing it, like washing or cleaning excessively, counting or checking things over and over, or repeating, collecting, arranging things, or other superstitious rituals?	NO	YES [compulsions]	4
	ARE H3 OR H4 CODED YES?	➡ NO	YES	
H5	Did you recognize that either these obsessive thoughts or these compulsive behaviors were excessive or unreasonable?	➡ NO	YES	5
H6	Did these obsessive thoughts and/or compulsive behaviors significantly interfere with your normal routine, occupational functioning, usual social activities, or relationships, or did they take more than one hour a day?	NO	YES O.C.D. CURRENT	6

M.I.N.I. 5.0.0 (July 1, 1999)   13

I. POSTTRAUMATIC STRESS DISORDER (optional)

(➡ MEANS : GO TO THE DIAGNOSTIC BOX, CIRCLE NO, AND MOVE TO THE NEXT MODULE)

I1	Have you ever experienced or witnessed or had to deal with an extremely traumatic event that included actual or threatened death or serious injury to you or someone else?		➡ NO	YES	1
	EXAMPLES OF TRAUMATIC EVENTS INCLUDE: SERIOUS ACCIDENTS, SEXUAL OR PHYSICAL ASSAULT, A TERRORIST ATTACK, BEING HELD HOSTAGE, KIDNAPPING, FIRE, DISCOVERING A BODY, SUDDEN DEATH OF SOMEONE CLOSE TO YOU, WAR, OR NATURAL DISASTER.				
I2	During the past month, have you re-experienced the event in a distressing way (such as, dreams, intense recollections, flashbacks or physical reactions)?		➡ NO	YES	2

I3	**In the past month:**				
	a	Have you avoided thinking about the event, or have you avoided things that remind you of the event?	NO	YES	3
	b	Have you had trouble recalling some important part of what happened?	NO	YES	4
	c	Have you become less interested in hobbies or social activities?	NO	YES	5
	d	Have you felt detached or estranged from others?	NO	YES	6
	e	Have you noticed that your feelings are numbed?	NO	YES	7
	f	Have you felt that your life will be shortened or that you will die sooner than other people?	NO	YES	8
		ARE 3 OR MORE I3 ANSWERS CODED YES?	➡ NO	YES	
I4	**In the past month:**				
	a	Have you had difficulty sleeping?	NO	YES	9
	b	Were you especially irritable or did you have outbursts of anger?	NO	YES	10
	c	Have you had difficulty concentrating?	NO	YES	11
	d	Were you nervous or constantly on your guard?	NO	YES	12
	e	Were you easily startled?	NO	YES	13
		ARE 2 OR MORE I4 ANSWERS CODED YES?	➡ NO	YES	

I5 During the past month, have these problems significantly interfered with your work or social activities, or caused significant distress?	14 **NO YES** *POSTTRAUMATIC STRESS DISORDER CURRENT*

J. ALCOHOL ABUSE AND DEPENDENCE

(➡ MEANS : GO TO THE DIAGNOSTIC BOXES, CIRCLE NO IN ALL DIAGNOSTIC BOXES, AND MOVE TO THE NEXT MODULE)

J1	In the past 12 months, have you had 3 or more alcoholic drinks within a 3 hour period on 3 or more occasions?	➡ NO	YES	1

J2   **In the past 12 months:**

a   Did you need to drink more in order to get the same effect that you got when you first started drinking?   NO   YES   2

b   When you cut down on drinking did your hands shake, did you sweat or feel agitated? Did you drink to avoid these symptoms or to avoid being hungover, for example, "the shakes", sweating or agitation?
IF YES TO EITHER, CODE YES.   NO·   YES   3

c   During the times when you drank alcohol, did you end up drinking more than you planned when you started?   NO   YES   4

d   Have you tried to reduce or stop drinking alcohol but failed?   NO   YES   5

e   On the days that you drank, did you spend substantial time in obtaining alcohol, drinking, or in recovering from the effects of alcohol?   NO   YES   6

f   Did you spend less time working, enjoying hobbies, or being with others because of your drinking?   NO   YES   7

g   Have you continued to drink even though you knew that the drinking caused you health or mental problems?   NO   YES   8

ARE 3 OR MORE **J2** ANSWERS CODED **YES**?

NO	➡ YES
ALCOHOL DEPENDENCE **CURRENT**	

J3   **In the past 12 months:**

a   Have you been intoxicated, high, or hungover more than once when you had other responsibilities at school, at work, or at home? Did this cause any problems? (CODE YES ONLY IF THIS CAUSED PROBLEMS.)   NO   YES   9

b   Were you intoxicated in any situation where you were physically at risk, for example, driving a car, riding a motorbike, using machinery, boating, etc.?   NO   YES   10

c   Did you have any legal problems because of your drinking, for example, an arrest or disorderly conduct?   NO   YES   11

d   Did you continue to drink even though your drinking caused problems with your family or other people?   NO   YES   12

ARE 1 OR MORE **J3** ANSWERS CODED **YES**?

NO	YES
ALCOHOL ABUSE **CURRENT**	

M.I.N.I. 5.0.0 (July 1, 1999)   15

K. NON-ALCOHOL PSYCHOACTIVE SUBSTANCE USE DISORDERS

(➡ MEANS : GO TO THE DIAGNOSTIC BOXES, CIRCLE NO IN ALL DIAGNOSTIC BOXES, AND MOVE TO THE NEXT MODULE)

K1	a	Now I am going to show you / read to you a list of street drugs or medicines. In the past 12 months, did you take any of these drugs more than once, to get high, to feel better, or to change your mood?	➡ NO YES

CIRCLE EACH DRUG TAKEN:

Stimulants: amphetamines, "speed", crystal meth, "rush", Dexedrine, Ritalin, diet pills.

Cocaine: snorting, IV, freebase, crack, "speedball".

Narcotics: heroin, morphine, Dilaudid, opium, Demerol, methadone, codeine, Percodan, Darvon.

Hallucinogens: LSD ("acid"), mescaline, peyote, PCP ("Angel Dust", "peace pill"), psilocybin, STP, "mushrooms", ecstasy, MDA, or MDMA.

Inhalants: "glue", ethyl chloride, nitrous oxide, ("laughing gas"), amyl or butyl nitrate ("poppers").

Marijuana: hashish ("hash"), THC, "pot", "grass", "weed", "reefer".

Tranquilizers: quaalude, Seconal ("reds"), Valium, Xanax, Librium, Ativan, Dalmane, Halcion, barbiturates, Miltown.

Miscellaneous: steroids, nonprescription sleep or diet pills. Any others?

SPECIFY MOST USED DRUG(S): _____

b   SPECIFY WHICH WILL BE EXPLORED IN CRITERIA BELOW:

IF CONCURRENT OR SEQUENTIAL POLYSUBSTANCE USE:

       EACH DRUG CLASS USED INDIVIDUALLY.   ☐

       MOST USED DRUG CLASS ONLY.   ☐

       ONLY ONE DRUG / DRUG CLASS HAS BEEN USED.   ☐

K2   Considering your use of (NAME THE DRUG / DRUG CLASS SELECTED), in the past 12 months:

a	Have you found that you needed to use more (NAME OF DRUG / DRUG CLASS SELECTED) to get the same effect that you did when you first started taking it?	NO	YES	1
b	When you reduced or stopped using (NAME OF DRUG / DRUG CLASS SELECTED), did you have withdrawal symptoms (aches, shaking, fever, weakness, diarrhea, nausea, sweating, heart pounding, difficulty sleeping, or feeling agitated, anxious, irritable, or depressed)? Did you use any drug(s) to keep yourself from getting sick (withdrawal symptoms) or so that you would feel better?	NO	YES	2
	IF YES TO EITHER, CODE YES.			
c	Have you often found that when you used (NAME OF DRUG / DRUG CLASS SELECTED), you ended up taking more than you thought you would?	NO	YES	3
d	Have you tried to reduce or stop taking (NAME OF DRUG / DRUG CLASS SELECTED) but failed?	NO	YES	4
e	On the days that you used (NAME OF DRUG / DRUG CLASS SELECTED), did you spend substantial time (>2 HOURS), obtaining, using or in recovering from the drug, or thinking about the drug?	NO	YES	5

M.I.N.I. 5.0.0 (July 1, 1999)   16

f Did you spend less time working, enjoying hobbies, or being with family or friends because of your drug use?   NO   YES   6

g Have you continued to use (NAME OF DRUG / DRUG CLASS SELECTED), even though it caused you health or mental problems?   NO   YES   7

ARE 3 OR MORE **K2** ANSWERS CODED **YES**?

SPECIFY DRUG(S): _____

> **NO**   → **YES**
>
> **DRUG DEPENDENCE CURRENT**

Considering your use of (NAME THE DRUG CLASS SELECTED), **in the past 12 months:**

K3 a Have you been intoxicated, high, or hungover from (NAME OF DRUG / DRUG CLASS SELECTED) more than once, when you had other responsibilities at school, at work, or at home? Did this cause any problem?   NO   YES   8

    (CODE **YES** ONLY IF THIS CAUSED PROBLEMS.)

  b Have you been high or intoxicated from (NAME OF DRUG / DRUG CLASS SELECTED) in any situation where you were physically at risk (for example, driving a car, riding a motorbike, using machinery, boating, etc.)?   NO   YES   9

  c Did you have any legal problems because of your drug use, for example, an arrest or disorderly conduct?   NO   YES   10

  d Did you continue to use (NAME OF DRUG / DRUG CLASS SELECTED), even though it caused problems with your family or other people?   NO   YES   11

ARE 1 OR MORE **K3** ANSWERS CODED **YES**?

SPECIFY DRUG(S): _____

> **NO**   **YES**
>
> **DRUG ABUSE CURRENT**

L. PSYCHOTIC DISORDERS

ASK FOR AN EXAMPLE OF EACH QUESTION ANSWERED POSITIVELY. CODE YES ONLY IF THE EXAMPLES CLEARLY SHOW A DISTORTION OF THOUGHT OR OF PERCEPTION OR IF THEY ARE NOT CULTURALLY APPROPRIATE. BEFORE CODING, INVESTIGATE WHETHER DELUSIONS QUALIFY AS "BIZARRE".

DELUSIONS ARE "BIZARRE" IF: CLEARLY IMPLAUSIBLE, ABSURD, NOT UNDERSTANDABLE, AND CANNOT DERIVE FROM ORDINARY LIFE EXPERIENCE.

HALLUCINATIONS ARE SCORED "BIZARRE" IF: A VOICE COMMENTS ON THE PERSON'S THOUGHTS OR BEHAVIOR, OR WHEN TWO OR MORE VOICES ARE CONVERSING WITH EACH OTHER.

Now I am going to ask you about unusual experiences that some people have.

					BIZARRE	
L1	a	Have you ever believed that people were spying on you, or that someone was plotting against you, or trying to hurt you? NOTE: ASK FOR EXAMPLES TO RULE OUT ACTUAL STALKING.	NO	YES	YES	1
	b	IF YES: do you currently believe these things?	NO	YES	YES ➡L6	2
L2	a	Have you ever believed that someone was reading your mind or could hear your thoughts, or that you could actually read someone's mind or hear what another person was thinking?	NO	YES	YES	3
	b	IF YES: do you currently believe these things?	NO	YES	YES ➡L6	4
L3	a	Have you ever believed that someone or some force outside of yourself put thoughts in your mind that were not your own, or made you act in a way that was not your usual self? Have you ever felt that you were possessed? CLINICIAN: ASK FOR EXAMPLES AND DISCOUNT ANY THAT ARE NOT PSYCHOTIC.	NO	YES	YES	5
	b	IF YES: do you currently believe these things?	NO	YES	YES ➡L6	6
L4	a	Have you ever believed that you were being sent special messages through the TV, radio, or newspaper, or that a person you did not personally know was particularly interested in you?	NO	YES	YES	7
	b	IF YES: do you currently believe these things?	NO	YES	YES ➡L6	8
L5	a	Have your relatives or friends ever considered any of your beliefs strange or unusual? INTERVIEWER: ASK FOR EXAMPLES. ONLY CODE YES IF THE EXAMPLES ARE CLEARLY DELUSIONAL IDEAS NOT EXPLORED IN QUESTIONS L1 TO L4, FOR EXAMPLE, SOMATIC OR RELIGIOUS DELUSIONS OR DELUSIONS OF GRANDIOSITY, JEALOUSY, GUILT, RUIN OR DESTITUTION, ETC.	NO	YES	YES	9
	b	IF YES: do they currently consider your beliefs strange?	NO	YES	YES	10
L6	a	Have you ever heard things other people couldn't hear, such as voices?	NO	YES		11
		HALLUCINATIONS ARE SCORED "BIZARRE" ONLY IF PATIENT ANSWERS YES TO THE FOLLOWING: IF YES: Did you hear a voice commenting on your thoughts or behavior or did you hear two or more voices talking to each other?			YES	
	b	IF YES: have you heard these things in the past month?	NO	YES	YES ➡L8b	12

MINI STRUCTURED INTERVIEW (continued)

L7 a Have you ever had visions when you were awake or have you ever seen things other people couldn't see?
CLINICIAN: CHECK TO SEE IF THESE ARE CULTURALLY INAPPROPRIATE.

NO   YES   13

b IF YES: have you seen these things in the past month?

NO   YES   14

CLINICIAN'S JUDGMENT

L8 b IS THE PATIENT CURRENTLY EXHIBITING INCOHERENCE, DISORGANIZED SPEECH, OR MARKED LOOSENING OF ASSOCIATIONS?

NO   YES   15

L9 b IS THE PATIENT CURRENTLY EXHIBITING DISORGANIZED OR CATATONIC BEHAVIOR?

NO   YES   16

L10 b ARE NEGATIVE SYMPTOMS OF SCHIZOPHRENIA, E.G. SIGNIFICANT AFFECTIVE FLATTENING, POVERTY OF SPEECH (ALOGIA) OR AN INABILITY TO INITIATE OR PERSIST IN GOAL-DIRECTED ACTIVITIES (AVOLITION), PROMINENT DURING THE INTERVIEW?

NO   YES   17

L11 ARE 1 OR MORE « b » QUESTIONS CODED YES BIZARRE?

OR

ARE 2 OR MORE « b » QUESTIONS CODED YES (RATHER THAN YES BIZARRE)?

NO	YES
PSYCHOTIC SYNDROME **CURRENT**	

L12 ARE 1 OR MORE « a » QUESTIONS CODED YES BIZARRE?

OR

ARE 2 OR MORE « a » QUESTIONS CODED YES (RATHER THAN YES BIZARRE)?

CHECK THAT THE TWO SYMPTOMS OCCURRED DURING THE SAME TIME PERIOD.

OR IS L11 CODED YES?

NO	YES	18
PSYCHOTIC SYNDROME **LIFETIME**		

L13 a IS L11 CODED YES AND IS EITHER

MAJOR DEPRESSIVE EPISODE, (CURRENT)
OR
MANIC EPISODE, (CURRENT OR PAST) CODED YES?

NO   YES

b IF L13a IS CODED YES:

You told me earlier that you had period(s) when you felt (depressed/high/persistently irritable).
Were the beliefs and experiences you just described (SYMPTOMS CODED YES FROM L1 b TO L7 b) restricted exclusively to times when you were feeling depressed/high/irritable?

NO	YES	19
MOOD DISORDER WITH PSYCHOTIC FEATURES **CURRENT**		

M. ANOREXIA NERVOSA

(➡ MEANS : GO TO THE DIAGNOSTIC BOX, CIRCLE NO, AND MOVE TO THE NEXT MODULE)

M1 a How tall are you?

☐.☐☐ ft. in.

☐ ☐☐ cm.

b. What was your lowest weight in the past 3 months?

☐ ☐☐ lbs.

☐ ☐☐ kgs.

c IS PATIENT'S WEIGHT LOWER THAN THE THRESHOLD CORRESPONDING TO HIS / HER HEIGHT? (SEE TABLE BELOW)   ➡ NO   YES

In the past 3 months:

M2 In spite of this low weight, have you tried not to gain weight?   ➡ NO   YES   1

M3 Have you feared gaining weight or becoming fat, even though you were underweight?   ➡ NO   YES   2

M4 a Have you considered yourself fat or that part of your body was too fat?   NO   YES   3

b Has your body weight or shape greatly influenced how you felt about yourself?   NO   YES   4

c Have you thought that your current low body weight was normal or excessive?   NO   YES   5

M5 ARE 1 OR MORE ITEMS FROM **M4** CODED **YES**?   ➡ NO   YES

M6 FOR WOMEN ONLY: During the last 3 months, did you miss all your menstrual periods when they were expected to occur (when you were not pregnant)?   ➡ NO   YES   6

FOR WOMEN: ARE **M5** AND **M6** CODED **YES**?

FOR MEN: IS **M5** CODED **YES**?

NO	YES
ANOREXIA NERVOSA **CURRENT**	

TABLE HEIGHT / WEIGHT THRESHOLD (height-without shoes; weight-without clothing)

Female Height/Weight													
ft/in	4'9	4'10	4'11	5'0	5'1	5'2	5'3	5'4	5'5	5'6	5'7	5'8	5'9	5'10
lbs.	84	85	86	87	89	92	94	97	99	102	104	107	110	112
cm	145	147	150	152	155	158	160	163	165	168	170	173	175	178
kgs	38	39	39	40	41	42	43	44	45	46	47	49	50	51

Male Height/Weight													
ft/in	5'1	5'2	5'3	5'4	5'5	5'6	5'7	5'8	5'9	5'10	5'11	6'0	6'1	6'2	6'3
lbs.	105	106	108	110	111	113	115	116	118	120	122	125	127	130	133
cm	155	156	160	163	165	168	170	173	175	178	180	183	185	188	191
kgs	47	48	49	50	51	51	52	53	54	55	56	57	58	59	61

The weight thresholds above are calculated as a 15% reduction below the normal range for the patient's height and gender as required by DSM-IV. This table reflects weights that are 15% lower than the low end of the normal distribution range in the Metropolitan Life Insurance Table of Weights.

N. BULIMIA NERVOSA

(➡ MEANS : GO TO THE DIAGNOSTIC BOXES, CIRCLE NO IN ALL DIAGNOSTIC BOXES, AND MOVE TO THE NEXT MODULE)

N1	In the past three months, did you have eating binges or times when you ate a very large amount of food within a 2-hour period?	➡ NO	YES	7
N2	In the last 3 months, did you have eating binges as often as twice a week?	➡ NO	YES	8
N3	During these binges, did you feel that your eating was out of control?	➡ NO	YES	9
N4	Did you do anything to compensate for, or to prevent a weight gain from these binges, like vomiting, fasting, exercising or taking laxatives, enemas, diuretics (fluid pills), or other medications?	➡ NO	YES	10
N5	Does your body weight or shape greatly influence how you feel about yourself?	➡ NO	YES	11
N6	DO THE PATIENT'S SYMPTOMS MEET CRITERIA FOR ANOREXIA NERVOSA?	NO ↓ Skip to N8	YES	
N7	Do these binges occur only when you are under (____lbs./kgs.)? (INTERVIEWER: WRITE IN THE ABOVE PARENTHESIS THE THRESHOLD WEIGHT FOR THIS PATIENT'S HEIGHT FROM THE HEIGHT / WEIGHT TABLE IN THE ANOREXIA NERVOSA MODULE.)	NO	YES	12

N8   IS N5 CODED YES AND N7 CODED NO OR SKIPPED?

> **NO   YES**
>
> *BULIMIA NERVOSA*
> **CURRENT**

IS N7 CODED YES?

> **NO   YES**
>
> *ANOREXIA NERVOSA*
> *Binge Eating/Purging Type*
> **CURRENT**

O. GENERALIZED ANXIETY DISORDER

(➡ MEANS : GO TO THE DIAGNOSTIC BOX, CIRCLE NO, AND MOVE TO THE NEXT MODULE)

O1	a	Have you worried excessively or been anxious about several things over the past 6 months?	➡ NO YES	1
	b	Are these worries present most days?	➡ NO YES	2
		IS THE PATIENT'S ANXIETY RESTRICTED EXCLUSIVELY TO, OR BETTER EXPLAINED BY, ANY DISORDER PRIOR TO THIS POINT?	NO YES	3
O2		Do you find it difficult to control the worries or do they interfere with your ability to focus on what you are doing?	➡ NO YES	4

O3   FOR THE FOLLOWING, CODE NO IF THE SYMPTOMS ARE CONFINED TO FEATURES OF ANY DISORDER EXPLORED PRIOR TO THIS POINT.

When you were anxious over the past 6 months, did you, most of the time:

a	Feel restless, keyed up or on edge?	NO YES	5
b	Feel tense?	NO YES	6
c	Feel tired, weak or exhausted easily?	NO YES	7
d	Have difficulty concentrating or find your mind going blank?	NO YES	8
e	Feel irritable?	NO YES	9
f	Have difficulty sleeping (difficulty falling asleep, waking up in the middle of the night, early morning wakening or sleeping excessively)?	NO YES	10

ARE 3 OR MORE O3 ANSWERS CODED YES?

> **NO   YES**
>
> *GENERALIZED ANXIETY DISORDER*
> **CURRENT**

MINI STRUCTURED INTERVIEW (continued)

REFERENCES

Sheehan DV, Lecrubier Y, Harnett-Sheehan K, Janavs J, Weiller E, Bonara LI, Keskiner A, Schinka J, Knapp E, Sheehan MF, Dunbar GC. Reliability and Validity of the MINI International Neuropsychiatric Interview (M.I.N.I.): According to the SCID-P. European Psychiatry. 1997; 12:232-241.

Lecrubier Y, Sheehan D, Weiller E, Amorim P, Bonora I, Sheehan K, Janavs J, Dunbar G. The MINI International Neuropsychiatric Interview (M.I.N.I.) A Short Diagnostic Structured Interview: Reliability and Validity According to the CIDI. European Psychiatry. 1997; 12: 224-231.

Sheehan DV, Lecrubier Y, Harnett-Sheehan K, Amorim P, Janavs J, Weiller E, Hergueta T, Baker R, Dunbar G: The Mini International Neuropsychiatric Interview (M.I.N.I.): The Development and Validation of a Structured Diagnostic Psychiatric Interview.. J. Clin Psychiatry, 1998;59(suppl 20):22-33.

Amorim P, Lecrubier Y, Weiller E, Hergueta T, Sheehan D: DSM-III-R Psychotic Disorders: procedural validity of the Mini International Neuropsychiatric Interview (M.I.N.I.). Concordance and causes for discordance with the CIDI. European Psychiatry. 1998: 13:26-34.

Translations	M.I.N.I. 4.4 or earlier versions	M.I.N.I. 4.6/5.0, M.I.N.I. Plus 4.6/5.0 and M.I.N.I. Screen 5.0:
Afrikaans	In preparation	
Arabic		Prof. Emsley
Basque		O. Osman, E. Al-Radi
Bengali		In preparation
Brazilian Portugese	P. Amorim	H. Banerjee, A. Banerjee
Bulgarian		P. Amorim
Catalan		Dr. Hranov
Chinese		In preparation
Croatian		L. Carroll, K-d Juang
Czech		In preparation
Danish	P. Bech	P. Zvlosky
Dutch/Flemish	E. Griez, K. Shruers, T. Overbeek, K. Demyttenaere	P. Bech, T. Schütze
English	D. Sheehan, J. Janavs, R. Baker, K. Harnett-Sheehan,	I. Van Vliet, H. Leroy, H. van Megen
	E. Knapp, M. Sheehan	D. Sheehan, R. Baker, J. Janavs, K. Harnett-Sheehan,
		M. Sheehan
Estonian		Dr. Shlik
Farsi/Persian		K. Khooshabi, A. Zomorodi
Finnish	M. Heikkinen, M. Lijeström, O. Tuominen	M. Heikkinen, M. Lijeström, O. Tuominen
French	Y. Lecrubier, E. Weiller, L. Bonora, P. Amorim, J.P. Lepine	Y. Lecrubier, E. Weiller, P. Amorim, T. Hergueta
German	I. v. Denffer, M. Ackenheil, R. Dietz-Bauer	G. Stotz, R. Dietz-Bauer, M. Ackenheil
Greek	S. Beratis	T. Calligas, S. Beratis
Gujarati		M. Patel, B. Patel
Hebrew	J. Zohar, Y. Sasson	R. Barda, I. Levinson
Hindi		C. Mittal, K. Batra, S. Gambhir
Hungarian	I. Bitter, J. Balazs	I. Bitter, J. Balazs
Icelandic		Prof. Petursson
Italian	L. Bonora, L. Conti, M. Piccinelli, M. Tansella, G. Cassano,	L. Conti, A. Rossi, P. Donda
	Y. Lecrubier, P. Donda, E. Weiller	
Japanese		H. Watanabe,T. Otsubo
Korean		In preparation
Latvian	V. Janavs, J. Janavs, I. Nagobads	V. Janavs, J. Janavs
Norwegian	G. Pedersen, S. Blomhoff	K.A. Leiknes , U. Malt, E. Malt, S. Leganger
Polish	M. Masiak, E. Jasiak	M. Masiak, E. Jasiak
Portuguese	P. Amorim	P. Amorim, T. Guterres
Punjabi		A. Gahunia, S. Gambhir
Romanian		O. Driga
Russian		A. Bystritsky, E. Selivra, M. Bystritsky
Serbian	I. Timotijevic	I. Timotijevic
Setswana		K. Ketlogetswe
Slovenian	M. Kocmur	M. Kocmur
Spanish	L. Ferrando, J. Bobes-Garcia, J. Gilbert-Rahola, Y. Lecrubier	L. Ferrando, L. Franco-Alfonso, M. Soto, J. Bobes-Garcia, O. Soto, L. Franco
Swedish	M. Waern,, S. Andersch, M. Humble	C. Allgulander, M. Waern, A. Brimse, M. Humble,
Turkish	T. Örnek, A. Keskiner, I. Vahip	T. Örnek, A. Keskiner
Urdu		A. Taj, S. Gambhir
Welsh		In preparation

A validation study of this instrument was made possible, in part, by grants from SmithKline Beecham and the European Commission.

The authors are grateful to Dr. Pauline Powers for her advice on the modules on Anorexia Nervosa and Bulimia.

M.I.N.I. 5.0.0 (July 1, 1999)   24

SHEEHAN PATIENT RATED ANXIETY SCALE

(reproduced with permission. ©1982 David V. Sheehan. All rights reserved.)

Instructions: Below is a list of problems and complaints that people sometimes have. Part 1 asks about how you have felt during THE PAST WEEK; Part 2 asks about how you feel RIGHT NOW. Mark only one box for each problem, and do not skip any items.

	Not At All	A Little	Moderately	Markedly	Extremely
Part 1: During the past week, how much did you suffer from...					
1. Difficulty in getting your breath, smothering, or overbreathing.					
2. Choking sensation or lump in throat.					
3. Skipping, racing, or pounding of your heart.					
4. Chest pain, pressure, or discomfort.					
5. Bouts of excessive sweating.					
6. Faintness, light-headedness, or dizzy spells.					
7. Sensation of rubbery or "jelly" legs.					
8. Feeling off balance or unsteady like you might fall.					
9. Nausea or stomach problems.					
10. Feeling that things around you are strange, unreal, foggy, or detached from you.					
11. Feeling outside or detached from part or all of your body, or a floating feeling.					
12. Tingling or numbness in parts of your body.					
13. Hot flashes or cold chills.					

SHEEHAN PATIENT RATED ANXIETY SCALE (continued)

	Not At All	A Little	Moderately	Markedly	Extremely
Part 1 (continued): During the past week, how much did you suffer from...					
14. Shaking or trembling.					
15. Having a fear that you are dying or that something terrible is about to happen.					
16. Feeling you are losing control or going insane.					
17. *SITUATIONAL ANXIETY ATTACK* Sudden anxiety attacks with 4 or more of the symptoms listed previously that occur when you are in or about to go into a situation that is likely, from your experience, to bring on an attack.					
18. *UNEXPECTED ANXIETY ATTACK* Sudden unexpected anxiety attacks with 4 or more symptoms (listed previously) that occur with little or no provocation (i.e., when you are NOT in a situation that is likely, from your experience, to bring on an attack).					
19. *UNEXPECTED LIMITED SYMPTOM ATTACK* Sudden unexpected spells with only one or two symptoms (listed previously) that occur with little or no provocation (i.e., when you are NOT in a situation that is likely, from your experience, to bring on an attack).					
20. *ANTICIPATORY ANXIETY EPISODE* Anxiety episodes that build up as you anticipate doing something that is likely, from your experience, to bring on anxiety that is more intense than most people experience in such situations.					
21. Avoiding situations because they frighten you.					

SHEEHAN PATIENT RATED ANXIETY SCALE (continued)

	Not At All	A Little	Moderately	Markedly	Extremely
Part 1 (continued): During the past week, how much did you suffer from...					
22. Being dependent on others.					
23. Tension and inability to relax.					
24. Anxiety, nervousness, restlessness.					
25. Spells of increased sensitivity to sound, light, or touch.					
26. Attacks of diarrhea.					
27. Worrying about your health too much.					
28. Feeling tired, weak, and exhausted easily.					
29. Headaches or pains in neck or head.					
30. Difficulty in falling asleep.					
31. Waking in the middle of the night, or restless sleep.					
32. Unexpected waves of depression occurring with little or no provocation.					
33. Emotions and moods going up and down a lot in response to changes around you.					
34. Recurrent and persistent ideas, thoughts, impulses, or images that are intrusive, unwanted, senseless, or repugnant.					
35. Having to repeat the same action in a ritual, e.g., checking, washing, counting repeatedly, when it's not really necessary.					

SHEEHAN PATIENT RATED ANXIETY SCALE (continued)

	Not At All	A Little	Moderately	Markedly	Extremely
Part 2: Right now, at this moment...					
1. Mouth drier than usual.					
2. Worried, preoccupied.					
3. Nervous, jittery, anxious, restless.					
4. Afraid, fearful.					
5. Tense, uptight.					
6. Shaky inside or out.					
7. Fluttery stomach.					
8. Warm all over.					
9. Sweaty palms.					
10. Rapid or heavy heart beat.					
11. Tremor of hands or legs.					

Not At All =0   A Little =1   Moderately =2   Markedly =3   Extremely =4

Add total for Part I and Part II separately. The average for Part I at first presentation of panic disorder is 57 ± 20. 37-77/standard deviation around mean. Scores below 25 are unusual in untreated panic disorder. The goal of treatment is a score lower than 15.

PART I

25-37	37-57	57-77	>77
mild	moderate	severe	very severe

PART II

0-10	11-25	26-44
mild	moderate	severe

TREATMENT OUTCOME PTSD SCALE (TOP-8)

Initials_____ ID#_____ Date_____ Visit #_____

Age_____ Sex_____ Race_____

The interviewer should identify which traumatic event is the most bothersome and then rate how much each symptom has troubled the subject during the past week.

Event: _____

1. Have you experienced painful images, thoughts or memories of the event which you could not get out of your mind even though you may have wanted to?   _____

   0 = not at all
   1 = mild: rarely and/or not bothersome
   2 = moderate: at least once a week and/or produces some distress
   3 = severe: at least 4 times per week or moderately distressing
   4 = extremely severe; daily or produces so much distress that patient cannot work or function socially

2. Does exposure to an event that reminds you of, or resembles the event, cause you to have any physical response (e.g., sweating, trembling, heart racing, nausea, hyperventilating, dizziness, etc.)?   _____

   0 = not at all
   1 = a little bit: infrequent or questionable
   2 = somewhat: mildly distressing
   3 = significantly: causes much distress
   4 = marked: very distressing; may have sought help because of the physical response (e.g., chest pain so severe that patient was sure he or she was having a heart attack)

3. Have you avoided places, people, conversations or activities that remind you of the event (e.g., movies, TV shows, certain places, meetings, funerals)?   _____

   0 = no avoidance
   1 = mild: of doubtful significance
   2 = moderate: definite avoidance of situations
   3 = severe: very uncomfortable and avoidance affects life in some way
   4 = extremely severe: house-bound, cannot go out to shops or restaurants, major functional restrictions

4. Have you experienced less interest (pleasure) in things that you used to enjoy?   _____

   0 = no loss of interest
   1 = one or two activities less pleasurable
   2 = several activities less pleasurable
   3 = most activities less pleasurable
   4 = almost all activities less pleasurable

5. Do you have less to do with other people than you used to?
   Do you feel estranged from other people?   _____

   0 = no problem
   1 = feels detached/estranged, but still normal degree of contact
       with others
   2 = sometimes avoids contact that would normally participate in
   3 = definitely and usually avoids people with whom would previously
       associate
   4 = absolutely refuses or actively avoids all social contact

6. Can you have warm feelings/feel close to others? Do you feel numb? _____

   0 = no problem
   1 = mild: of questionable significance
   2 = moderate: some difficulty expressing feelings
   3 = severe: definite problems with expressing feelings
   4 = very severe: have no feelings, feels numb most of the time

7. Do you have to stay on guard? Are you watchful? Do you feel
   on edge? Do you have to sit with your back to the wall?   _____

   0 = no problem
   1 = mild: occasional/not disruptive
   2 = moderate: causes discomfort/feels on edge or watchful in some
       situations
   3 = severe: causes discomfort/feels on edge or watchful in most
       situations
   4 = very severe: causes extreme discomfort and/or alters life
       (feels constantly on guard/socially impaired because of
       hypervigilance)

8. Do you startle easily? Do you have a tendency to jump? Is this a
   problem after unexpected noise, or if you hear or see something that
   reminds you of the trauma?   _____

   0 = no problem
   1 = mild: occasional but not disruptive
   2 = moderate: causes definite discomfort or an exaggerated startle
       response at least every two weeks
   3 = severe: happens more than once a week
   4 = extremely severe: so bad that patient cannot function at work or
       socially

TOTAL SCORE   _____

DAVIDSON TRAUMA SCALE
by Jonathan R. T. Davidson, M.D

Name: _John Brown_   Age: __34__   Sex: ☑ Male   ○ Female

Date: __06/ 10 /96__

Please identify the trauma that is most disturbing to you.

Car accident — two close friends were seriously injured

Each of the following questions asks you about a specific symptom. For each question, consider how often in the last week the symptom troubled you and how severe it was. In the two boxes beside each question, write a number from 0 – 4 to indicate the frequency and severity of the symptom.

FREQUENCY	SEVERITY
0 = Not at all	0 = Not at all distressing
1 = Once only	1 = Minimally distressing
2 = 2-3 times	2 = Moderately distressing
3 = 4-6 times	3 = Markedly distressing
4 = Every day	4 = Extremely distressing

	Frequency	Severity
1. Have you ever had painful images, memories, or thoughts of the event?	4	3
2. Have you ever had distressing dreams of the event?	4	3
3. Have you been upset by something that reminded you of the event?	2	1
4. Have you been avoiding any thoughts or feelings about the event?	3	4
5. Have you been avoiding doing things or going into situations that remind you of the event?	2	2
6. Have you had difficulty enjoying things?	4	4

FLORIDA YALE-BROWN OBSESSIVE COMPULSIVE SCALE (FLY-BOCS)

Developed by Wayne K. Goodman, M.D., Department of Psychiatry, University of Florida College of Medicine; Steven A. Rasmussen, M.D., Lawrence H. Price, M.D., Department of Psychiatry, Brown University School of Medicine.

General Instructions

This rating scale is designed to rate the severity and type of symptoms in patients with obsessive compulsive disorder (OCD). In general, the items depend on the patient's report; however, the final rating is based on the clinical judgement of the interviewer. Rate the characteristics of each item during the prior week up until and including the time of the interview. Scores should reflect the average (mean) occurrence of each item for the entire week.

This rating scale is intended for use as a semi-structured interview. The interviewer should assess the items in the listed order and use the questions provided. However, the interviewer is free to ask additional questions for purposes of clarification. If the patient volunteers information at any time during the interview, that information will be considered. Ratings should be based primarily on reports and observations gained during the interview. If you judge that the information being provided is grossly inaccurate, then the reliability of the patient is in doubt and should be noted accordingly at the end of the interview (item 19).

Additional information supplied by others (e.g., spouse or parent) may be included in a determination of the ratings only if it is judged that (1) such information is essential to adequately assessing symptom severity *and* (2) consistent week-to-week reporting can be ensured by having the same informant(s) present for each rating session.

Before proceeding with the questions, define "obsessions" and "compulsions" for the patient as follows:

> *"OBSESSIONS are unwelcome and distressing ideas, thoughts, images or impulses that repeatedly enter your mind. They may seem to occur against your will. They may be repugnant to you, you may recognize them as senseless, and they may not fit your personality."*

> *"COMPULSIONS, on the other hand, are behaviors or acts that you feel driven to perform although you may recognize them as senseless or excessive. At times, you may try to resist doing them but this may prove difficult. You may experience anxiety that does not diminish until the behavior is completed."*

> *"Let me give you some examples of obsessions and compulsions."*

> *"An example of an obsession is: the recurrent thought or impulse to do serious physical harm to your children even though you never would."*

> *"An example of a compulsion is: the need to repeatedly check appliances, water faucets, and the lock on the front door before you can leave the house. While most*

FLORIDA YALE-BROWN OBSESSIVE COMPULSIVE SCALE (FLY-BOCS) (continued)

compulsions are observable behaviors, some are unobservable mental acts, such as silent checking or having to recite nonsense phrases to yourself each time you have a bad thought."

"Do you have any questions about what these words mean?" [If not, proceed.]

On repeated testing it is not always necessary to re-read these definitions and examples as long as it can be established that the patient understands them. It may be sufficient to remind the patient that obsessions are the thoughts or concerns and compulsions are the things you feel driven to do, including covert mental acts.

Have the patient enumerate current obsessions and compulsions in order to generate a list of target symptoms. Use the FLY-BOCS Symptom Checklist as an aid for identifying current symptoms. It is also useful to identify and be aware of past symptoms since they may re-appear during subsequent ratings. Once the current types of obsessions and compulsions are identified, organize and list them on the Target Symptoms form according to clinically convenient distinctions (e.g., divide target compulsions into checking and washing). Describe salient features of the symptoms so that they can be more easily tracked (e.g., in addition to listing checking, specify what the patient checks for). Be sure to indicate which are the most prominent symptoms; i.e., those that will be the major focus of assessment. Note, however, that the final score for each item should reflect a composite rating of all of the patient's obsessions or compulsions.

The rater must ascertain whether reported behaviors are bona fide symptoms of OCD and not symptoms of another disorder, such as Simple Phobia or a Paraphilia. The differential diagnosis between certain complex motor tics and certain compulsions (e.g., involving touching) may be difficult or impossible. In such cases, it is particularly important to provide explicit descriptions of the target symptoms and to be consistent in subsequent ratings. Separate assessment of tic severity with a tic rating instrument may be necessary in such cases. Some of the items listed on the FLY-BOCS Symptom Checklist, such as trichotillomania, are currently classified in DSM-IV as symptoms of an Impulse Control Disorder. It should be noted that the suitability of the FLY-BOCS for use in disorders other than DSM-IV-defined OCD has yet to be established. However, when using the FLY-BOCS to rate severity of symptoms not strictly classified under OCD (e.g., trichotillomania) in a patient who otherwise meets criteria for OCD, it has been our practice to administer the FLY-BOCS twice: once for conventional obsessive-compulsive symptoms, and a second time for putative OCD-related phenomena. In this fashion separate FLY-BOCS scores are generated for severity of OCD and severity of other symptoms in which the relationship to OCD is still unsettled.

On repeated testing, review and, if necessary, revise target obsessions prior to rating item 1. Do likewise for compulsions prior to rating item 6.

The total FLY-BOCS score is the sum of items 1-10 (excluding 1b and 6b), whereas the obsession and compulsion subtotals are the sums of items 1-5 (excluding 1b) and 6-10 (excluding 6b), respectively.

FLORIDA YALE-BROWN OBSESSIVE COMPULSIVE SCALE (FLY-BOCS) (continued)

Name_____ Date_____

Check all that apply, but clearly mark the principal symptoms with a "P."
(Rater must ascertain whether reported behaviors are bona fide symptoms of OCD, and not symptoms of another disorder such as Simple Phobia or Hypochondriasis. Items marked with an asterisk (*) may or may not be OCD phenomena.)

Current	Past	
		AGGRESSIVE OBSESSIONS
_____	_____	Fear might harm self
_____	_____	Fear might harm others
_____	_____	Violent or horrific images
_____	_____	Fear of blurting out obscenities or insults
_____	_____	Fear of doing something else embarrassing*
_____	_____	Fear will act on unwanted impulses (e.g., to stab friend)
_____	_____	Fear will steal things
_____	_____	Fear will harm others because not careful enough (e.g., hit/run MVA)
_____	_____	Fear will be responsible for something else terrible happening (e.g., fire, burglary)
_____	_____	Other_____
		CONTAMINATION OBSESSIONS
_____	_____	Concerns or disgust with bodily waste or secretions (e.g., urine, feces, saliva)
_____	_____	Concern with dirt or germs
_____	_____	Excessive concern with environmental contaminants (e.g., asbestos, radiation, toxic waste)
_____	_____	Excessive concern with household items (e.g., cleansers, solvents)
_____	_____	Excessive concern with animals (e.g., insects)
_____	_____	Bothered by sticky substances or residues
_____	_____	Concerned will get ill because of contaminant
_____	_____	Concerned will get others ill by spreading contaminant (Aggressive)
_____	_____	No concern with consequences of contamination other than how it might feel
_____	_____	Other_____

FLORIDA YALE-BROWN OBSESSIVE COMPULSIVE SCALE (FLY-BOCS)
(continued)

Current	Past	
		SEXUAL OBSESSIONS
_____	_____	Forbidden or perverse sexual thoughts, images, or impulses
_____	_____	Content involves children or incest
_____	_____	Content involves homosexuality*
_____	_____	Sexual behavior toward others (Aggressive)*
_____	_____	Other_____

HOARDING/SAVING OBSESSIONS

| _____ | _____ | [distinguish from hobbies and concern with objects of monetary or sentimental value] |
| _____ | _____ | Other_____ |

RELIGIOUS OBSESSIONS (Scrupulosity)

_____	_____	Concerned with sacrilege and blasphemy
_____	_____	Excess concern with right/wrong, morality
_____	_____	Other_____

OBSESSION WITH NEED FOR SYMMETRY OR EXACTNESS

| _____ | _____ | Accompanied by magical thinking (e.g., concerned that mother will have accident unless things are in the right place) |
| _____ | _____ | Not accompanied by magical thinking |

MISCELLANEOUS OBSESSIONS

_____	_____	Need to know or remember
_____	_____	Fear of saying certain things
_____	_____	Fear of not saying just the right thing
_____	_____	Fear of losing things
_____	_____	Intrusive (non-violent) images
_____	_____	Intrusive nonsense sounds, words, or music
_____	_____	Bothered by certain sounds/noises*
_____	_____	Lucky/unlucky numbers
_____	_____	Colors with special significance
_____	_____	Superstitious fears
_____	_____	Other_____

FLORIDA YALE-BROWN OBSESSIVE COMPULSIVE SCALE (FLY-BOCS) (continued)

Current   **Past**

SOMATIC OBSESSIONS

_____   _____   Concern with illness or disease*

_____   _____   Excessive concern with body part or aspect of appearance (e.g., dysmorphophobia)*

_____   _____   Other_____

CLEANING/WASHING COMPULSIONS

_____   _____   Excessive or ritualized handwashing

_____   _____   Excessive or ritualized showering, bathing, toothbrushing, grooming

_____   _____   Involves cleaning of household items or other inanimate objects

_____   _____   Other measures to prevent or remove contact with contaminants

_____   _____   Other_____

CHECKING COMPULSIONS

_____   _____   Checking locks, stove, appliances, etc

_____   _____   Checking that did not/will not harm others

_____   _____   Checking that did not/will not harm self

_____   _____   Checking that nothing terrible did/will happen

_____   _____   Checking that did not make mistake

_____   _____   Checking tied to somatic obsessions

_____   _____   Other_____

REPEATING RITUALS

_____   _____   Re-reading or re-writing

_____   _____   Need to repeat routine activities (e.g., in/out door, up/down from chair)

_____   _____   Other_____

COUNTING COMPULSIONS

_____   _____   _____

ORDERING/ARRANGING COMPULSIONS

_____   _____   _____

FLORIDA YALE-BROWN OBSESSIVE COMPULSIVE SCALE (FLY-BOCS) (continued)

Current	Past	
		HOARDING/COLLECTING COMPULSIONS [distinguish from hobbies and concern with objects of monetary or sentimental value (e.g., carefully reads junk mail, piles up old newspapers, sorts through garbage, collects useless objects)]

MISCELLANEOUS COMPULSIONS

Current	Past	
		Mental rituals (other than checking/counting)
		Excessive list making
		Need to tell, ask, or confess
		Need to touch, tap, or rub*
		Rituals involving blinking or staring*
		Measures (not checking) to prevent: harm to self_____; harm to others_____; terrible consequences_____
		Ritualized eating behaviors*
		Superstitious behaviors
		Trichotillomania*
		Other self-damaging or self-mutilating behaviors*
		Other_____

FLORIDA YALE-BROWN OBSESSIVE COMPULSIVE SCALE (FLY-BOCS) (continued)

Name_____ Date_____

TARGET SYMPTOM LIST

OBSESSIONS:

1. _____
_____
2. _____
_____
3. _____
_____
_____
_____

COMPULSIONS:

1. _____
_____
2. _____
_____
3. _____
_____
_____

AVOIDANCE:

1. _____
_____
2. _____
_____
3. _____
_____
_____

FLORIDA YALE-BROWN OBSESSIVE COMPULSIVE SCALE (FLY-BOCS) (continued)

"I am now going to ask several questions about your obsessive thoughts." [Make specific reference to the patient's target obsessions.]

1. <u>TIME OCCUPIED BY OBSESSIVE THOUGHTS</u>

    Q: How much of your time is occupied by obsessive thoughts? [When obsessions occur as brief, intermittent intrusions, it may be difficult to assess time occupied by them in terms of total hours. In such cases, estimate time by determining how frequently they occur. Consider both the number of times the intrusions occur and how many hours of the day are affected. Ask:] How frequently do the obsessive thoughts occur? [Be sure to exclude ruminations and preoccupations which, unlike obsessions, are ego-syntonic and rational (but exaggerated).]

    > 0 = None
    >
    > 1 = Mild, less than 1 hr/day or occasional intrusion
    >
    > 2 = Moderate, 1 to 3 hrs/day or frequent intrusion
    >
    > 3 = Severe, greater than 3 and up to 8 hrs/day or very frequent intrusion
    >
    > 4 = Extreme, greater than 8 hrs/day or near constant intrusion

1b. <u>OBSESSION-FREE INTERVAL</u> (not included in total score)

    Q: On the average, what is the longest number of consecutive waking hours per day that you are completely free of obsessive thoughts? [If necessary, ask:] What is the longest block of time in which obsessive thoughts are absent?

    > 0 = No symptoms
    >
    > 1 = Long symptom-free interval, more than 8 consecutive hrs/day symptom-free
    >
    > 2 = Moderately long symptom-free interval, more than 3 and up to 8 consecutive hrs/day symptom-free
    >
    > 3 = Short symptom-free interval, from 1 to 3 consecutive hrs/day symptom-free
    >
    > 4 = Extremely short symptom-free interval, less than 1 consecutive hr/day symptom-free

FLORIDA YALE-BROWN OBSESSIVE COMPULSIVE SCALE (FLY-BOCS) (continued)

2. INTERFERENCE DUE TO OBSESSIVE THOUGHTS

    Q: How much do your obsessive thoughts interfere with your social or work (or role) functioning? Is there anything that you don't do because of them? [If currently not working determine how much performance would be affected if patient were employed.]

        0 = None

        1 = Mild, slight interference with social or occupational activities, but overall performance not impaired

        2 = Moderate, definite interference with social or occupational performance, but still manageable

        3 = Severe, causes substantial impairment in social or occupational performance

        4 = Extreme, incapacitating

3. DISTRESS ASSOCIATED WITH OBSESSIVE THOUGHTS

    Q: How much distress do your obsessive thoughts cause you? [In most cases, distress is equated with anxiety; however, patients may report that their obsessions are "disturbing" but deny "anxiety." Only rate anxiety that seems triggered by obsessions, not generalized anxiety or anxiety associated with other conditions.]

        0 = None

        1 = Mild, not too disturbing

        2 = Moderate, disturbing, but still manageable

        3 = Severe, very disturbing

        4 = Extreme, near constant and disabling distress

4. RESISTANCE AGAINST OBSESSIONS

    Q: How much of an effort do you make to resist the obsessive thoughts? How often do you try to disregard or turn your attention away from these thoughts as they enter your mind? [Only rate effort made to resist, not success or failure in actually controlling the obsessions. How much the patient resists the obsessions may or may not correlate with his ability to control them. Note that this item does not directly measure the severity of the intrusive thoughts; rather it rates a manifestation of health, i.e., the effort the patient makes to counteract the obsessions by means other than avoidance or the performance of compulsions. Thus, the more the patient tries to resist, the less impaired is this aspect of his functioning. There are "active" and "passive" forms of resistance. Patients in behavioral therapy may be encouraged to counteract their obsessive symptoms by not struggling against them (e.g., "just let the thoughts come"; passive opposition) or by intentionally bringing on the disturbing thoughts. For the purposes of this item, consider use of these behavioral techniques as forms of resistance.

FLY-BOCS

FLORIDA YALE-BROWN OBSESSIVE COMPULSIVE SCALE (FLY-BOCS) (continued)

If the obsessions are minimal, the patient may not feel the need to resist them. In such cases, a rating of "0" should be given.]

    0 = Makes an effort to always resist, or symptoms so minimal doesn't need to actively resist

    1 = Tries to resist most of the time

    2 = Makes some effort to resist

    3 = Yields to all obsessions without attempting to control them, but does so with some reluctance

    4 = Completely and willingly yields to all obsessions

5.   <u>DEGREE OF CONTROL OVER OBSESSIVE THOUGHTS</u>

    Q: How much control do you have over your obsessive thoughts? How successful are you in stopping or diverting your obsessive thinking? Can you dismiss them? [In contrast to the preceding item on resistance, the ability of the patient to control his obsessions is more closely related to the severity of the intrusive thoughts.]

        0 = Complete control

        1 = Much control, usually able to stop or divert obsessions with some effort and concentration

        2 = Moderate control, sometimes able to stop or divert obsessions

        3 = Little control, rarely successful in stopping or dismissing obsessions, can only divert attention with difficulty

        4 = No control, experienced as completely involuntary, rarely able to even momentarily alter obsessive thinking

"The next several questions are about your compulsive behaviors." [Make specific reference to the patient's target compulsions.]

6.   <u>TIME SPENT PERFORMING COMPULSIVE BEHAVIORS</u>

    Q: How much time do you spend performing compulsive behaviors? [When rituals involving activities of daily living are chiefly present, ask:] How much longer than most people does it take to complete routine activities because of your rituals? [When compulsions occur as brief, intermittent behaviors, it may be difficult to assess time spent performing them in terms of total hours. In such cases, estimate time by determining how frequently they are performed. Consider both the number of times compulsions are performed and how many hours of the day are affected. Count separate occurrences of compulsive behaviors, not number of repetitions; e.g., a patient who goes into the bathroom 20 different times a day to wash his hands 5 times very quickly, performs compulsions 20 times a day, not 5 or $5 \times 20 = 100$. Ask:] How frequently do you perform compulsions? [In most cases compulsions are observable behaviors (e.g., handwashing), but some compulsions are covert (e.g., silent checking).]

FLORIDA YALE-BROWN OBSESSIVE COMPULSIVE SCALE (FLY-BOCS) (continued)

    0 = None

    1 = Mild (spends less than 1 hr/day performing compulsions), or occasional performance of compulsive behaviors

    2 = Moderate (spends from 1 to 3 hrs/day performing compulsions), or frequent performance of compulsive behaviors

    3 = Severe (spends more than 3 and up to 8 hrs/day performing compulsions), or very frequent performance of compulsive behaviors

    4 = Extreme (spends more than 8 hrs/day performing compulsions), or near constant performance of compulsive behaviors (too numerous to count)

6b.   COMPULSION-FREE INTERVAL (not included in total score)

    Q: On the average, what is the longest number of consecutive waking hours per day that you are completely free of compulsive behavior? [If necessary, ask:] What is the longest block of time in which compulsions are absent?

        0 = No symptoms

        1 = Long symptom-free interval, more than 8 consecutive hrs/day symptom-free

        2 = Moderately long symptom-free interval, more than 3 and up to 8 consecutive hrs/day symptom-free

        3 = Short symptom-free interval, from 1 to 3 consecutive hrs/day symptom-free

        4 = Extremely short symptom-free interval, less than 1 consecutive hr/day symptom-free

7.   INTERFERENCE DUE TO COMPULSIVE BEHAVIORS

    Q: How much do your compulsive behaviors interfere with your social or work (or role) functioning? Is there anything that you don't do because of the compulsions? [If currently not working determine how much performance would be affected if patient were employed.]

        0 = None

        1 = Mild, slight interference with social or occupational activities, but overall performance not impaired

        2 = Moderate, definite interference with social or occupational performance, but still manageable

        3 = Severe, causes substantial impairment in social or occupational performance

        4 = Extreme, incapacitating

FLORIDA YALE-BROWN OBSESSIVE COMPULSIVE SCALE (FLY-BOCS) (continued)

8. DISTRESS ASSOCIATED WITH COMPULSIVE BEHAVIOR

    Q: How would you feel if prevented from performing your compulsion(s)? [Pause]. How anxious would you become? [Rate degree of distress patient would experience if performance of the compulsion were suddenly interrupted without reassurance offered. In most, but not all cases, performing compulsions reduces anxiety. If, in the judgement of the interviewer, anxiety is actually reduced by preventing compulsions in the manner described above, then ask:] How anxious do you get while performing compulsions until you are satisfied they are completed?

    0 = None

    1 = Mild, only slightly anxious if compulsions prevented, or only slight anxiety during performance of compulsions

    2 = Moderate, reports that anxiety would mount but remain manageable if compulsions prevented, or that anxiety increases but remains manageable during performance of compulsions

    3 = Severe, prominent and very disturbing increase in anxiety if compulsions interrupted, or prominent and very disturbing increase in anxiety during performance of compulsions

    4 = Extreme, incapacitating anxiety from any intervention aimed at modifying activity, or incapacitating anxiety develops during performance of compulsions

9. RESISTANCE AGAINST COMPULSIONS

    Q: How much of an effort do you make to resist the compulsions? [Only rate effort made to resist, not success or failure in actually controlling the compulsions. How much the patient resists the compulsions may or may not correlate with his ability to control them. Note that this item does not directly measure the severity of the compulsions; rather it rates a manifestation of health, i.e., the effort the patient makes to counteract the compulsions. Thus, the more the patient tries to resist, the less impaired is this aspect of his functioning. If the compulsions are minimal, the patient may not feel the need to resist them. In such cases, a rating of "0" should be given.]

    0 = Makes an effort to always resist, or symptoms so minimal doesn't need to actively resist

    1 = Tries to resist most of the time

    2 = Makes some effort to resist

    3 = Yields to almost all compulsions without attempting to control them, but does so with some reluctance

    4 = Completely and willingly yields to all compulsions

10. <u>DEGREE OF CONTROL OVER COMPULSIVE BEHAVIOR</u>

 Q: How strong is the drive to perform the compulsive behavior? [Pause]. How much control do you have over the compulsions? [In contrast to the preceding item on resistance, the ability of the patient to control his compulsions is more closely related to the severity of the compulsions.]

        0 = Complete control

        1 = Much control, experiences pressure to perform the behavior but usually able to exercise voluntary control over it

        2 = Moderate control, strong pressure to perform behavior, can control it only with difficulty

        3 = Little control, very strong drive to perform behavior, must be carried to completion, can only delay with difficulty

        4 = No control, drive to perform behavior experienced as completely involuntary and overpowering, rarely able to even momentarily delay activity

FLORIDA YALE-BROWN OBSESSIVE COMPULSIVE SCALE (FLY-BOCS) (continued)

FLY-BOCS TOTAL (add items 1-10) ☐

PATIENT NAME_____ DATE_____

PATIENT ID_____ RATER_____

		None	Mild	Moderate	Severe	Extreme
1.	TIME SPENT ON OBSESSIONS	0	1	2	3	4

		No Symptoms	Long	Moderately Long	Short	Extremely Short
1b.	OBSESSION-FREE INTERVAL (do not add to subtotal or total score)	0	1	2	3	4

2.	INTERFERENCE FROM OBSESSIONS	0	1	2	3	4

3.	DISTRESS OF OBSESSIONS	0	1	2	3	4

		Always Resists				Completely Yields
4.	RESISTANCE	0	1	2	3	4

		Complete Control	Much Control	Moderate Control	Little Control	No Control
5.	CONTROL OVER OBSESSIONS	0	1	2	3	4

OBSESSION SUBTOTAL (add items 1-5) ☐

FLORIDA YALE-BROWN OBSESSIVE COMPULSIVE SCALE (FLY-BOCS) (continued)

		None	Mild	Moderate	Severe	Extreme
6.	TIME SPENT ON COMPULSIONS	None 0	Mild 1	Moderate 2	Severe 3	Extreme 4

		No Symptoms	Long	Moderately Long	Short	Extremely Short
6b.	COMPULSION-FREE INTERVAL (do not add to subtotal or total score)	No Symptoms 0	Long 1	Moderately Long 2	Short 3	Extremely Short 4

7.	INTERFERENCE FROM COMPULSIONS	0	1	2	3	4
8.	DISTRESS OF COMPULSIONS	0	1	2	3	4

		Always Resists				Completely Yields
9.	RESISTANCE	Always Resists 0	1	2	3	Completely Yields 4

		Complete Control	Much Control	Moderate Control	Little Control	No Control
10.	CONTROL OVER COMPULSIONS	Complete Control 0	Much Control 1	Moderate Control 2	Little Control 3	No Control 4

COMPULSION SUBTOTAL (add items 6-10)

Additional information regarding the development, use, and psychometric properties of this scale can be found in Goodman WK, Price LH, Rasmussen SA, et al.: The Yale-Brown Obsessive Compulsive Scale (YBOCS): Part 1. Development, use, and reliability. *Arch Gen Psychiatry* (46:1006-1011, 1989), and Goodman WK, Price LH, Rasmussen SA, et al.: The Yale-Brown Obsessive Compulsive Scale (Y-BOCS): Part 2. Validity. *Arch Gen Psychiatry* (46:1012-1016, 1989).

Index

Antidepressants. *See also* Monoamine oxidase
  inhibitors; Selective serotonin reuptake
  inhibitors; Tricyclic antidepressants
  insomnia and, 43
  miscellaneous types of, 91–103
  pregnancy/lactation and, 162, **163**
  treatment of
    alcohol abuse and dependence and, 49
    Alzheimer's disease and, 67
    anorexia nervosa and, 58
    bipolar disorder and, 37, 40
    bulimia nervosa and, 60
    generalized anxiety disorder and, 15, 16
    major depressive disorder and, 27, **29**
    panic disorder and, 5, 7
    posttraumatic stress disorder and, 13
    social anxiety disorder and, 20
Antidiabetic agents, and monoamine oxidase
  inhibitors, **90**
Antihistamines. *See also* Nonsedating antihistamines
  drug interactions and, **124**
  extrapyramidal side effects and, 147–149
Antihypertensives, and insomnia, **42**
Antineoplastics, and insomnia, **42**
Antipsychotics. *See also* Clozapine; Olanzapine;
  Quetiapine; Risperidone
  Alzheimer's disease and, 65, 67
  atypical subgroup of, 137–144
  bipolar disorder and, 37, 40
  cocaine abuse and dependence and, 52
  drug interactions and, **79, 85, 105, 108**
  obsessive-compulsive disorder and, 9
  pregnancy and, **163**
  schizophrenia and, 72
  typical subgroup of, 130–136
Anxiety disorders
  adolescent depression and, 30
  elderly and, **166**
  overview of and pharmacotherapy for, 3–21
  resources on, 171
  Sheehan Patient Rated Anxiety Scale and,
    232–235
Anxiety Disorders Association of America, 171
Anxiolytics, and anorexia nervosa, 57. *See also*
  Benzodiazepines; Buspirone; Meprobamate
Aprobarbital (Alurate), **123.** *See also* Barbiturates
Area Agency on Aging, 171
Aricept. *See* Donepezil
Artane. *See* Trihexyphenidyl
Asendin. *See* Amoxapine
Aspirin, and drug interactions, **111**
Asthma, and pharmacotherapy for depression, **29**
Ativan. *See* Lorazepam
AUDIT (Alcohol Use Disorders Identification
  Test), 49

B

Barbiturates
  dosing guidelines for, 125
  drug interactions and, **79, 90, 108,** 123, **124,
    127, 133**
  efficacy of, 123
  overview of oral therapy, **122**
  pharmacokinetics of, **123**
  side effects of, 125
  warnings and precautions, 125
Beck Depression Inventory (BDI), **24**
Behavior
  Alzheimer's disease and, 65, 67
  obsessive-compulsive disorder and, **9**
Behavioral therapy, and anorexia nervosa, 57.
  See also Cognitive-behavioral therapy;
  Psychotherapy
Benadryl. *See* Diphenhydramine
Benzodiazepines. *See also* Alprazolam; Clonazepam; Lorazepam
  alcohol abuse and dependence and, 49–50
  bipolar disorder and, 37
  comparative features of, **114**
  dosing guidelines for, 117
  drug interactions and, **85, 99, 108,** 115, **116**
  efficacy of, 115
  generalized anxiety disorder and, 15–16
  insomnia and, 43
  overview of therapy, **113**
  panic disorder and, 5, 7
  posttraumatic stress disorder and, 14
  pregnancy and, **163**
  schizophrenia and, 72
  side effects of, 115
  social anxiety disorder and, 20
  SSRI initiation period and, 86
  warnings and precautions, 116–117
Benzoylecgonine, and cocaine abuse, 51
Benztropine (Cogentin), 147. *See also* Anticholinergics
Beta-blockers
  drug interactions and, **85, 90, 124**
  extrapyramidal side effects and, 150
  posttraumatic stress disorder and, 14
Bethanechol, **153, 156**
Binge eating, 58
Biperiden, 145, 147
Bipolar disorder
  diagnosis of, 35, **36**
  differentiating features of subtypes, **34**
  epidemiology of, 34
  pathophysiology of, 34
  pregnancy and treatment of, **164**
  presentation of, 34–35
  referrals for, 35
  treatment of, 36–40, 104–112, **164**
Blessed Dementia Scale, 63
Body temperature. *See* Hyperthermia; Hypothermia

Clozapine (Clozaril). *See also* Antipsychotics
dosing guidelines, 139
drug interactions and, **138**
efficacy of, 138
overview of therapy, **137**
pharmacokinetics of, 136, 137
schizophrenia and, 72, 73, 138
side effects of, 138
warnings and precautions, 138–139
Clozaril. *See* Clozapine
Clozaril Patient Management System, 139
Cocaine abuse and dependence
diagnosis of, 51
epidemiology of, 50–51
pathophysiology of, 51
presentation of, 51
referrals for, 51
treatment of, 52
Cocaine Anonymous, 174
Cogentin. *See* Benztropine
Cognex. *See* Tacrine
Cognitive-behavioral therapy (CBT). *See also*
Behavioral therapy; Psychotherapy
bulimia nervosa and, 60
obsessive-compulsive disorder and, 8
panic disorder and, 5
Cognitive enhancers
cholinesterase inhibitors, 152–154
donepezil, 155–156
ergoloid mesylates, 151
Combination therapy
obsessive-compulsive disorder and, 9
psychotic depression and, 135
Comorbidity, and psychiatric disorders. *See also*
Medical conditions
adolescent depression and, 30
anorexia nervosa and, 55
definition of, 177
generalized anxiety disorder and, 14
major depressive disorder and, 27, **29**
panic disorder and, 3
posttraumatic stress disorder and, 12, 13
social anxiety disorder and, 18
Compazine. *See* Prochlorperazine
Compliance, with pharmacotherapy. *See also*
Patients
bipolar disorder and, 36–37
major depressive disorder and, 27
schizophrenia and, 70, 72
Compulsions, and obsessive-compulsive disorder,
7, 9
Corticosteroids, and drug interactions, **124**
Cyclosporin-A, **119**
Cylert. *See* Pemoline
Cytochrome P450 system (CYP450), 177

D

Daily living, Alzheimer's disease and activities
of, 62
Dalmane. *See* Flurazepam
Delirium tremens, 48
Delusions
Alzheimer's disease and, 62
definition of, 178
Dementia
dementia of the Alzheimer's type, 61–67
pharmacotherapy for depression and, **29**
Depakene. *See* Valproic acid
Depakote. *See* Valproic acid
Depression. *See also* Adolescent depression;
Major depressive disorder
elderly and
epidemiology of, 31
presentation of, 31
treatment of, 31–32, **166**
generalized anxiety disorder and, 14
pregnancy and, 162
resources on, 172–173
Depression/Awareness, Recognition and Treatment, 172
Desipramine (Norpramin). *See also* Tricyclic
antidepressants
cocaine abuse and, 52
comparative features of, **78**
depression in elderly and, 31
Desyrel. *See* Trazodone
Dexedrine. *See* Dextroamphetamine
Dextroamphetamine (Dexedrine), 158
Diagnosis, of psychiatric disorders. *See also*
Differential diagnosis
adolescent depression, 30
alcohol abuse and dependence, 48–49
Alzheimer's disease, 62–63, **64**
anorexia nervosa, 56–57
bipolar disorder, 35
bulimia nervosa, 59
cocaine abuse and dependence, 51
dysthymic disorder, 32, **33**
generalized anxiety disorder, 15
insomnia, 41–42
major depressive disorder, 24–25
obsessive-compulsive disorder, 8, **9**
opiate abuse and dependence, 53
panic disorder, 4–5
posttraumatic stress disorder, 12
schizophrenia, 69–70
social anxiety disorder, 18–20
somatization disorder, 44–45
*Diagnostic and Statistical Manual of Mental
Disorders*, fourth edition (DSM-IV,
American Psychiatric Association), 24
Diazepam (Valium). *See also* Benzodiazepines
comparative features of, **114**
drug interactions and, **97, 111**

G

General Health Questionnaire (GHQ), **24**
Generalized anxiety disorder (GAD)
  diagnosis of, 15
  epidemiology of, 14
  pathophysiology of, 14
  pharmacotherapy for depression and, **29**
  presentation of, 14
  referrals for, 15
  treatment of, 15–17
Genetics. *See also* Family
  obsessive-compulsive disorder and, 7
  panic disorder and, 3
  schizophrenia and, 68
Geriatric Depression Scale (GDS), **24**
Glaucoma
  antipsychotics and, **135**
  pharmacotherapy for depression and, **29**
Guanabenz, 54
Guanethidine, **79**
Guanfacine, 54

H

Halcion. *See* Triazolam
Haldol. *See* Haloperidol
Hallucinations, 178
Haloperidol (Haldol). *See also* Antipsychotics
  comparative features of, **131**
  drug interactions and, **79**, **85**, **99**, **119**
  side effects of, **134**
Hamilton Rating Scale for Depression (HAM-D),
  24
Head trauma, and pharmacotherapy for depression, **29**
Health care system. *See also* Medical conditions;
  Primary care and primary care physicians
  panic disorder and excessive use of services,
  3
  reasons for undertreatment of depression and,
  22
  somatoform disorders and, 44
  tobacco-related diseases and, 52
Hepatic impairment, and antipsychotics, **135**.
  See also Side effects
Hepatitis screening tests, 53
Hormones, and insomnia, **42**. *See also* Endo-
  crine disorders; Thyroid hormone
Hypertensive crisis, and monoamine oxidase
  inhibitors, 91
Hyperthermia
  anticholinergics and, 146–147
  antipsychotics and, **135**
Hypnotic agents, and insomnia, 43. *See also*
  Nonbarbiturate hypnotics; Sedative-
  hypnotics
Hypomania
  bipolar disorder and, 35, 36
  Mini Structured Interview and, 216–217
Hypothermia, and antipsychotics, **135**

I

Imipramine (Tofranil). *See also* Tricyclic antidepressants
  comparative features of, **78**
  drug interactions and, **129**
Incidence, of Alzheimer's disease, 61. *See also*
  Prevalence
Infectious diseases, and depression, 26
Insomnia
  benzodiazepines and, 115
  diagnosis of, 41–42
  elderly and, **166**
  epidemiology of, 41
  pathophysiology of, 41
  presentation of, 41
  referrals for, 43
  resources on, 173–174
  treatment of, 43, 166
Inventory for Depressive Symptomatology (IDS),
  24
Iodide salts, **105**
Isocarboxazid (Marplan), 88. *See also* Monoamine oxidase inhibitors
Itraconazole, **119**

J

Japanese ethnicity, and olanzapine, 139
Jaundice, and antipsychotics, 134
Jewish ethnicity, and clozapine, 138

K

Kemadrin. *See* Procyclidine
Ketoconazole, and drug interactions, **138**, **141**,
  156
Klonopin. *See* Clonazepam

L

LAAM (ORLAAM), and opiate abuse, 54
Laboratory tests
  Alzheimer's disease and, **64**
  anorexia nervosa and, **56**
  antipsychotics and false-positive, 132
  bulimia nervosa and, 59
  schizophrenia and, 69
Lactation, and quetiapine, 142. *See also* Pregnancy
Lamotrigine, **111**
Levodopa
  drug interactions and, **79**, **116**, **146**
  insomnia and, **42**
Librium. *See* Chlordiazepoxide
Liebowitz Social Anxiety Scale, 20, 208
Life expectancy, and Alzheimer's disease, 61
Lithium
  bipolar disorder and, 37, 40, 104–106
  dosing and monitoring guidelines for, 106
  drug interactions and, **85**, **105**, **108**, **133**
  efficacy of, 104–105

Lithium *(continued)*
    obsessive-compulsive disorder and, 9
    overview of therapy, **104**
    posttraumatic stress disorder and, 14
    pregnancy and, **163**
    side effects of, 106
    warnings and precautions, 106
Liver function tests (LFTs), 179
Lofexidine, 54
Lorazepam (Ativan), **114**. *See also* Benzodiaze-
    pines
Loxapine (Loxitane), **131.** *See also* Antipsychotics
Loxitane. *See* Loxapine
Ludiomil. *See* Maprotiline
Luvox. *See* Fluvoxamine

M

Macrolide antimicrobials, and drug interactions,
    108, 116
Maintenance therapy
    lithium and, 106
    methadone and opiate abuse, 54
    mood stabilization and, 40
    schizophrenia and, 72–73
Major depressive disorder. *See also* Depression
    diagnosis of, 24–25
    epidemiology of, 22–23
    Mini Structured Interview and, 212–213
    pathophysiology of, 23
    pregnancy and treatment of, **164**
    presentation of, 23
    reasons for undertreatment of, **22**
    referrals for, 26
    treatment of, 26–29, **164**
Mania and manic episodes
    adolescent depression and, 30
    bipolar disorder and, 35, 36, **38**
    elderly and, **166**
    major depressive disorder and, 23
    Mini Structured Interview and, 216–217
MAOIs. *See* Monoamine oxidase inhibitors
Maprotiline (Ludiomil). *See also* Tricyclic antide-
    pressants
    comparative features of, **78**
    lactation and, 81
    seizure disorders and, 81
Marplan. *See* Isocarboxazid
Mebaral. *See* Mephobarbital
Medical conditions. *See also* Comorbidity; Health
    care system
    alcohol abuse and dependence and, 48–49
    anorexia nervosa and, 57
    cocaine abuse and dependence and, 51
    comorbidity with psychiatric disorders and,
        25, **26**, **29**, 35
    differential diagnosis of psychiatric disorders
        and, 5, 63
    opiate abuse and dependence and, 53

Medications, insomnia caused by, **42**. *See also*
    Pharmacotherapy
Mellaril. *See* Thioridazine
Memory, and Alzheimer's disease, 62
Meperidine, and drug interactions, **90, 133**
Mephobarbital (Mebaral), **123.** *See also* Barbi-
    turates
Meprobamate (Equanil, Miltown)
    dosing guidelines for, 121
    drug interactions and, 120
    efficacy of, 120
    pharmacokinetics of, 120
    side effects of, 120
    warnings and precautions, 120–21
Mesoridazine (Serentil), **131.** *See also* Antipsy-
    chotics
Methadone (Dolophine) therapy, 54
Methyldopa, **105**
Methylphenidate (Ritalin), 158
Metronidazole, and drug interactions, **105, 124**
Michigan Alcoholism Screening Test (MAST), 49
Miltown. *See* Meprobamate
Mini International Neuropsychiatric Interview
    (MINI)
    alcohol abuse and dependence and, 49
    Alzheimer's disease and, 63
    anorexia nervosa and, 56
    bipolar disorder and, 35
    bulimia nervosa and, 59
    dysthymic disorder and, 32
    generalized anxiety disorder and, 15
    major depressive disorder and, 24
    obsessive-compulsive disorder and, 8
    panic disorder and, 4
    posttraumatic stress disorder and, 12
    social anxiety disorder and, 20
    text of, 209–231
Mini Mental State Examination (MMSE)
    Alzheimer's disease and, 63, 156
    definition of, 179
Mirtazapine (Remeron)
    comparative features of, **92**
    dosing guidelines for, 97
    drug interactions and, 96, **97**
    efficacy of, 96
    major depressive disorder and, 27
    overview of therapy, **96**
    side effects of, 97
    warning and precautions, 97
Moban. *See* Molindone
Molindone (Moban), **131.** *See also* Antipsy-
    chotics
Monitoring. *See* Plasma-level monitoring
Monoamine oxidase inhibitors (MAOIs)
    bipolar disorder and, 40
    bulimia nervosa and, 60
    depression in elderly and, 32
    dosing guidelines for, 91

Psychiatric disorders, and pharmacotherapy
(continued)
    eating disorders, 55–60
    mood disorders, 22–46
    treatment recommendations for elderly and,
        166
Psychosis. *See also* Schizophrenia
    treatment of in elderly, **166**
Psychotherapy. *See also* Behavioral therapy;
        Cognitive-behavioral therapy
    anorexia nervosa and, 57
    cocaine abuse and dependence and, 52
    somatization disorder and, 46
Public health
    Alzheimer's disease and, 61
    depression in the elderly and, 31–32
Purging subtype, of bulimia nervosa, 58–59

Q

Quazepam (Doral), **114.** *See also* Benzodiaze-
        pines
Quetiapine (Seroquel). *See also* Antipsychotics
    Alzheimer's disease and, 67
    dosing guidelines for, 142
    drug interactions and, **141**
    efficacy of, 142
    overview of therapy, **137**
    pharmacokinetics of, 136–137, 141
    schizophrenia and, 72, 73, 142
    side effects of, 142
    warnings and precautions, 142
Quinidine
    drug interactions and, **79**, **124**, **156**
    insomnia and, **42**

R

Ranitidine, **116**
Rapid-cycling bipolar disorder, 37, 40
Rapid neuroleptization, 72
Recovery, Incorporated, 173
Referrals, for psychiatric conditions
    Alzheimer's disease, 64
    anorexia nervosa, 57
    bipolar disorder, 35
    bulimia nervosa, 59–60
    cocaine abuse and dependence, 51
    dysthymic disorder, 33
    generalized anxiety disorder, 15
    insomnia, 43
    major depressive disorder, 26
    nicotine abuse and dependence, 52
    obsessive-compulsive disorder, 8
    opiate abuse, 54
    panic disorder, 5
    posttraumatic stress disorder, 12
    schizophrenia, 70
    social anxiety disorder, 20
    somatization disorder, 45

Relapse, and pharmacotherapy
    Alzheimer's disease and, 67
    obsessive-compulsive disorder and, 10
    social anxiety disorder and, 20
Remeron. *See* Mirtazapine
Renal impairment, and antipsychotics, 135
Resources, on pharmacotherapy for psychiatric
        disorders
    Alzheimer's disease, 170–171
    anxiety disorders, 171
    depression and mood disorders, 172–173
    general mental health, 169
    sleep disorders, 173–174
    substance use disorders, 174
Restoril. *See* Temazepam
Restricting subtype, of anorexia nervosa, 56
ReVia. *See* Naltrexone
Rifampin, and drug interactions, **116**, **124**, **140**
Risk factors
    for Alzheimer's disease, **61**
    for depression, 22, **23**
Risperdal. *See* Risperidone
Risperidone (Risperdal). *See also* Antipsychotics
    Alzheimer's disease and, 67
    dosing guidelines and, 144
    drug interactions and, **138**, 143
    efficacy of, 143
    overview of therapy, **137**
    pharmacokinetics of, 136, 143
    schizophrenia and, 72, 73, 143
    side effects of, 143
    warnings and precautions, 143
Ritalin. *See* Methylphenidate

S

Sandoz Clinical Assessment Geriatric Rating
        Scale, 151
Schizophrenia
    clozapine and, 138
    delusions and, 62
    diagnosis of, 69–70
    epidemiology of, 68
    pathophysiology of, 68
    pregnancy and treatment of, **164**
    presentation of, 68–69
    quetiapine and, 142
    referrals for, 70
    resources on, 173
    treatment of, 70–73, **164**
Secobarbital (Seconal), **123.** *See also* Barbitu-
        rates
Seconal. *See* Secobarbital
Sedative-hypnotics. *See also* Hypnotic agents
    barbiturates, 122–125
    nonbarbiturate hypnotics, 125–127
    zolpidem, 128–129
Seizures and seizure threshold
    antipsychotics and, 135
    bupropion and, 95

Seizures and seizure threshold *(continued)*
  pharmacotherapy for depression and, **29**
  tricyclic antidepressants and, 81
Selective serotonin reuptake inhibitors (SSRIs)
  adolescent depression and, 31
  Alzheimer's disease and, 67
  bipolar disorder and, 37, 40
  bulimia nervosa and, 60
  clozapine and, 137
  comparative features of, **83**
  depression in elderly and, 32
  dosing guidelines for, 87–88
  drug interactions and, **79**, 84, **85**, **90**, **105**,
    108, **138**
  dysthymic disorder and, 33
  efficacy of, 84
  major depressive disorder and, 27
  obsessive-compulsive disorder and, 9, **11**
  overview of therapy, **82**
  panic disorder and, 7
  pharmacokinetics of, **84**
  posttraumatic stress disorder and, 13
  pregnancy and, 162, **163**
  side effects of, 86
  social anxiety disorder and, 20
  somatization disorder and, 46
  warnings and precautions, 86
Selegiline (Eldepryl), and Alzheimer's disease,
    65, 156–157
Self-help groups
  cocaine abuse and dependence, 51, 52
  opiate abuse and dependence, 54
Serax. *See* Oxazepam
Serentil. *See* Mesoridazine
Seroquel. *See* Quetiapine
Serotonin syndrome
  definition of, 181
  selective serotonin reuptake inhibitors and, 84
Sertraline (Zoloft). *See also* Selective serotonin
    reuptake inhibitors
  comparative features of, **83**
  dosing guidelines for, 87
  obsessive-compulsive disorder and, **11**
  panic disorder and, 5
  pharmacokinetics of, **84**
Serzone. *See* Nefazodone
Seven-symptom screening test, for somatization
    disorder, **45**
Sexual dysfunction
  antipsychotics and, 134
  bupropion and, 93–94
  selective serotonin reuptake inhibitors and, 86
  trazodone and priapism, 101
Sheehan Patient Rated Anxiety Scale, 4, 232–235
Short Portable Mental Status Questionnaire, 63
Side effects, of pharmacotherapy. *See also*
    Agranulocytosis; Dosage-related toxic psy-
    chosis; Extrapyramidal side effects; Hepatic
    impairment; Therapeutic index

Side effects, of pharmacotherapy *(continued)*
  anorexia nervosa and psychotropic drug-
    induced, 57
  bipolar disorder and, 37
  elderly and treatment recommendations, 166
  of specific drugs
    amantadine, 149–150
    antipsychotics, 72, 73, **130**, 133–34
    barbiturates, **122**, **124**
    benzodiazepines, 7, **113**, 115
    bupropion, **93**, **96**
    buspirone, 119
    carbamazepine, **107**, 109
    donezepil, 155–156
    ergoloid mesylates, 151
    lithium, **104**, 106
    meprobamate, 120
    mirtazapine, 97
    monoamine oxidase inhibitors, **88**, 89
    naltrexone, 50
    nefazodone, 98–99
    nonbarbiturate hypnotics, 127
    olanzapine, 140
    quetiapine, 142
    risperidone, 143
    selective serotonin reuptake inhibitors, **82**,
      86
    selegiline, 157
    tacrine, **152**, 153
    trazodone, **100**, 101
    tricyclic antidepressants, 31, **77**, 80–81
    valproic acid, **110**, 112
    venlafaxine, **102**, 103
    zolpidem, **128**, 129
Sinequan. *See* Doxepin
Situationally bound and situationally predisposed
    panic attacks, 4–5
Sleep disorders. *See* Insomnia
Sleep hygiene, 41, 43
Sleep log, 42
Smoking. *See also* Nicotine
  olanzapine and, 139
  tobacco-related diseases and, 52
Social anxiety disorder
  common fears and sources of avoidance in,
    19
  definition of, 17
  diagnosis of, 18–20
  epidemiology of, 18
  Mini Structured Interview and, 220
  pathophysiology of, 18
  presentation of, 18
  referrals for, 20
  subtypes of, **17**
  treatment of, 20, **21**
Somatic symptoms
  major depressive disorder and, 23, 24
  panic disorder and, 4
Somatization disorder
  diagnosis of, 44–45

Z

Zidovudine, **111**
Zoloft. *See* Sertraline
Zolpidem (Ambien)
    dosage guidelines for, 129
    drug interactions and, 128, **129**
    efficacy of, 128
    insomnia and, 43, 128
    overview of therapy, **128**
    side effects of, 129
    warnings and precautions, 129
Zung Self-Rating Depression Scale (ZSRDS), **24**
Zyban. *See* Bupropion
Zyprexa. *See* Olanzapine